Lt. Col. W. S. Codrington's
KNOW YOUR HORSE
in health and disease
A Revision

by

PETER GRAY, M.V.B., M.R.C.V.S.

J. A. ALLEN
London

British Library Cataloguing in Publication Data

Codrington, W. S.
  Know your horse. — 7th ed.
  I. Title   II. Gray, Peter
  636.1089

  ISBN 0851315445

First published 1955 by Max Reinhardt
by J. A. Allen & Co. in 1963
Revised edition 1966
Reprinted 1968
Reprinted 1971
Reprinted 1972
Revised edition 1974
Reprinted 1975
Reprinted 1976
Reprinted 1978
Reprinted 1979
Reprinted 1981
Reprinted 1984
Reprinted 1986
Reprinted 1987
Revised edition 1992
Reprinted 1996

Published in Great Britain in 1992 by
J. A. Allen & Company Limited,
1, Lower Grosvenor Place, Buckingham Palace Road,
London, SW1W 0EL

Typeset in Hong Kong by Setrite Typesetters Ltd.
Printed in Hong Kong by Dah Hua Printing Co. Ltd.

Illustrations by Maggie Raynor
Designed by Nancy Lawrence

Contents

1   The Normal Body

To appreciate disease it is important to have an understanding of the normal animal body and the way it works. With this end in view it is proposed to devote the first part of this book to a simple and brief explanation of the anatomy and functions of the body.

The horse's body is divided into a head, a neck, a trunk, four limbs and a tail. The head and neck have a great deal of movement at the end of the more rigid trunk which gives attachment to the limbs. The head contains the brain and special sense organs (eyes, ears, nose and taste buds), and for efficient use of these, mobility is needed. The ability to move the head and neck is also important because it is through the mouth, equipped with teeth and mobile lips, that the horse ingests his food and water; through the nostrils he inhales air. The mouth is linked to the stomach through the gullet (oesophagus), the nostrils to the lungs through the windpipe (trachea).

The body, or trunk, is divided into two compartments. The front compartment, or chest cavity, formed outwardly by the ribs, houses the lungs and heart, while the rear compartment, housed within the abdominal muscles and pelvis, contains the stomach, bowels, liver, kidneys, bladder, spleen and various glands. These cavities are completely separated from each other by a sheet of muscle, attached to the ribs, known as the diaphragm.

The skeleton gives support and shape to the body. It is made up of a large number of bones joined together at joints which are bound by ligaments. For our purposes the important joints are in the limbs, because these are the most likely to be injured.

Limb Joints

The end of each long bone is dense, to withstand the effect of concussion taken by a joint. This explains why fractures occur more often in the

1

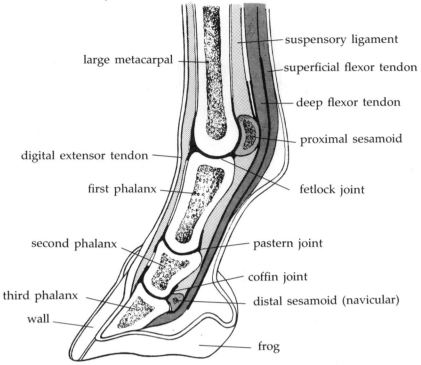

large metacarpal

suspensory ligament

superficial flexor tendon

deep flexor tendon

proximal sesamoid

digital extensor tendon

first phalanx

fetlock joint

second phalanx

pastern joint

coffin joint

third phalanx

distal sesamoid (navicular)

wall

frog

Cross section of the forelimb below the knee

shafts of long bones — which are hollow and weaker, especially in young horses.

The *articular surfaces* — the bone ends that meet in a joint — are covered by a layer of cartilage, a substance having greater elasticity than bone. Its function is to absorb concussion and reduce the chance of fracture.

Ligaments attach the bones to each other at the joint.

The *joint capsule*, consisting of an outer ligamentous portion and a synovial membrane, is responsible for binding the joint and producing the joint oil, *synovia*, which lubricates the articulating ends.

Although the skeleton forms the framework of the body, posture could not be maintained and movement could not occur without the *muscular system*. Muscles connect bones to each other and, in so doing, generate movement and give additional support to numerous joints.

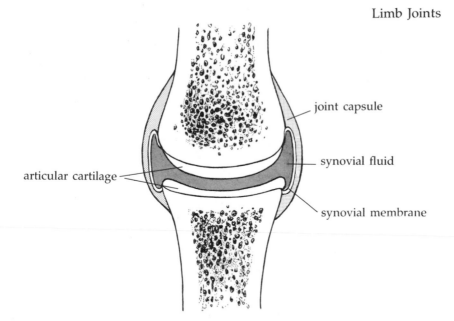

Anatomy of a joint

Contraction of the muscles is what creates the movement; this occuring through intervening joints. There is also interaction of joints in the horse. Consider how flexion of the hock causes the stifle and fetlock to become flexed too.

Throughout the limbs the muscles are distinguished as flexors and extensors, depending on their action. Flexor muscles bend the limbs while extensors project them forward when the animal is in flight. Abductors and adductors move the limbs in or away from a straight line. While a horse is resting, the muscles, and their sinewy extensions — the tendons — form a vital part of the stay apparatus which stabilises the joints and enables the animal to rest while standing. This facility permitted the horse in a wild environment to sleep on his feet — ready to flee a predator if the need arose.

Each limb muscle consists of a fleshy belly made up of red and white muscle fibres which are highly elastic and contractile, and a lower tendon consisting of fibrous tissue which attaches the belly to the bone and transmits the pull during contraction. The tendon is only fractionally elastic in comparison with the muscle belly, and this is part of the reason why tendon injury is so complicated.

Nowadays muscle fibres are classed according to type, which are basically differentiated through function. There are quick and slow contracting fibres, for speed and for strength. Slow fibres are used in lifting, quick fibres for acceleration. While these fibre types tend to be mixed in muscle, it is the predominance of one over the other that decides the type of athlete, be they endurance or short distance in nature.

All muscle operates under the control of nerves, which come from the brain via the spinal cord. Impulses are transmitted along the nerves to effect the movement required for ambulation. Inevitably this means that when an animal is walking or trotting there is alternate stimulation of flexors and extensors continually.

The Foot

Because of its intrinsic importance a more detailed description of the foot will be given. Its parts are divided thus:

    a. The skeleton of the foot
    b. The sensitive foot
    c. The insensitive foot.

a. The skeleton of the foot is made up of:

The Third Phalanx (Pedal or Coffin Bone)

This bone resembles the hoof in shape but is much smaller. It occupies only a portion of the cavity within the hoof.

The Accessory (or Lateral) Cartilages

These are elastic structures emanating from the wings of the pedal bone. They act as shock absorbers, assisting the elasticity of the foot as a whole. Under certain circumstances they become ossified − the condition known as side bone.

The Digital (Pedal or Plantar) Cushion

Lying between the two lateral cartilages is a mass of fibrous elastic tissue, situated between the undersurface of the pedal bone and the

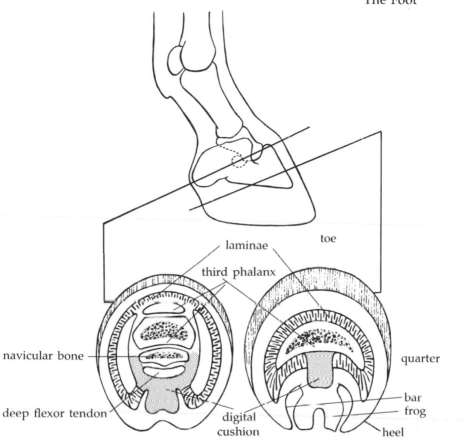

Cross section of foot at two levels

frog. It has a poor blood supply and is not very sensitive, but acts as one of the chief shock-absorbing structures of the foot. It lies beneath the deep digital flexor tendon and rests on the horny frog, unable to expand forward to any extent due to the pedal bone. It extends back to the bulbs of the heel and out to the lateral cartilages under the walls of the hoof.

The Navicular Bone (or Distal Sesamoid)

This is a small shuttle-shaped bone situated at the back of the pedal bone over which the deep flexor tendon passes before being attached to the pedal bone. It acts as a fulcrum to the tendon.

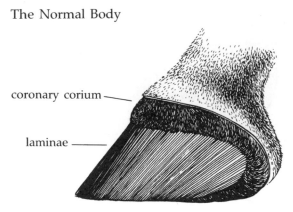

coronary corium —

laminae ———

Corium of foot

b. The sensitive foot is made up of:

The Coronary Band or Cushion

This encircles the coronet from one heel to the other situated at the junction of the wall and skin. It produces horn cells for the growth of the hoof.

The Corium of the Foot

The *laminar corium* covers the outer surface of the pedal bone. It corresponds with the inside of the hoof wall in being provided with about 600 leaves, called sensitive laminae. These interlock with the insensitive laminae of the hoof wall and hold the pedal bone in position. Covering the lower surface of the pedal bone is the *corium* of the *sole* (or sensitive sole), and covering the undersurface of the plantar cushion is the *corium* of the *frog* (or sensitive frog). These components of the corium merge with one another and are well supplied with blood vessels and nerves. They provide nourishment for the production of the horny parts of the wall, sole and frog.

The Perioplic Ring

Situated around the hoof, above the coronary band, this secretes a layer of waterproof varnish which covers the wall. Its purpose is to prevent moisture loss and accompanying shrinkage of the hoof and splitting of the wall.

c. The insensitive foot or hoof is modified skin composed of practically the same material as the horns and claws of other animals and is made up of:

The Wall

This is the part which can be seen when the foot is on the ground. It is composed of dense horn and covered by a layer of horny scales which give the surface a glossy appearance and help protect the wall from evaporation. On its inside are numerous leaves which interlock with similar leaves on the sensitive foot. The wall is arbitrarily divided into toe, quarters and heels.

The Bars

At the heels the wall turns inwards and forwards to form the bars which act as a reinforcement to prevent the wall contracting. The angles at which the walls and bars meet are termed the buttresses.

The Sole

This is the ground surface of the hoof. It provides protection for the foot and acts as a shock absorber. The sole meets the wall at the white line, a layer of softer horn uniting the two. This line is of great importance to the farrier because it indicates the distinction between sensitive and insensitive parts of the foot. As it delineates the thickness of the wall it is a guide to the positioning of nails when shoeing.

The Frog

This is a V-shaped structure interposed between the bars. It is made up of spongy horn which consists of about 50 per cent water. Its function is to absorb concussion and assist circulation to the structures of the foot.

2   The Body Systems

The systems of the body all operate interdependently. For study purposes, they are each approached as distinct entities, taken in the following sequence.

The Circulation

The circulatory system consists of the heart and all the blood vessels. The heart is a hollow muscular organ situated in the chest cavity. It is in fact a pump which sends the blood around the body, in what may be described as a closed circuit of pipes. The heart is divided into four separate compartments — two *atria* and two *ventricles*. The circulation is described in the *Circulatory system* diagram.

Blood from the lower right chamber of the heart — the right ventricle — is conveyed to the lungs where it is oxygenated and then returned to the left upper chamber — the left atrium — from whence it passes into the left ventricle. From the left ventricle it is conveyed all over the body in the *arteries*. Within the tissues, the arteries repeatedly branch and decrease in size as they go from the heart, until they are eventually only visible with the aid of a microscope. They then run into *capillaries* which follow through to the formation of *veins*, which in turn convey depleted blood back to the right atrium and thence into the right ventricle.

Blood, in general, does not come into direct contact with tissue cells except in the liver and spleen. At the level of the capillaries *plasma* constituents exude through the fine walls of the vessels into the tissue spaces. Tissue cells are bathed in a fluid called *interstitial fluid* which is derived from blood and approximates blood plasma in composition. This fluid is responsible for the nourishment of cells and also assists in the return of waste materials to the general circulation.

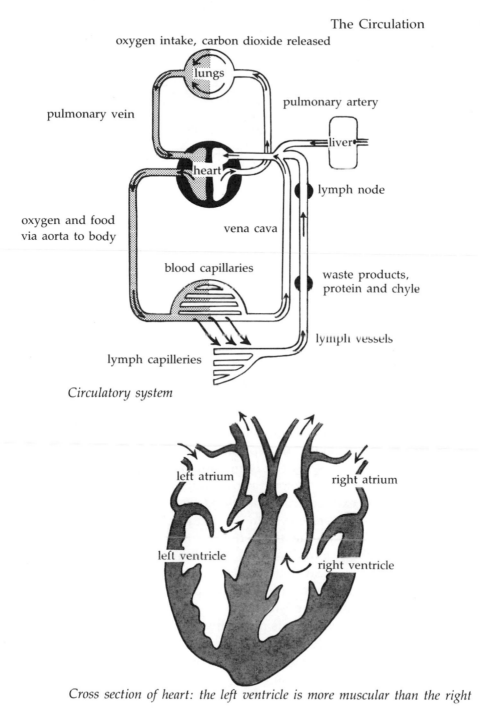

oxygen intake, carbon dioxide released

lungs

pulmonary vein

pulmonary artery

liver

heart

lymph node

oxygen and food
via aorta to body

vena cava

blood capillaries

waste products,
protein and chyle

lymph vessels

lymph capilleries

Circulatory system

left atrium

right atrium

left ventricle

right ventricle

Cross section of heart: the left ventricle is more muscular than the right

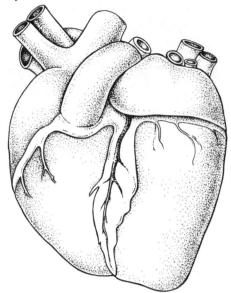

Outside of the heart showing the major blood vessels

Some of the fluid is returned to the vascular system through the *lymphatic system*, which is a system of thin-walled vessels existing only on the venous side of the circulation. It carries its content to entrances into the major veins in front of the heart. Most protein molecules are too large to be absorbed back into blood capillaries and find their way into lymph vessels. Also the absorption of fats and other nutrients from the bowel in digestion is via the lymphatic system, giving the fluid − known as *chyle* − a milky colour at this stage.

Once lymph has exuded from the blood vessels across the interstitial spaces into its own separate system its circulation is no longer aided by the pumping action of the heart. Its flow is influenced by the squeezing action of general body muscles, and lymph vessels are provided with *valves* − as are veins − so that the flow is unidirectional and space is left behind for the exudation of more lymph.

Lymph is similar in composition to blood plasma except that it is lower in certain proteins. It is normally a clear watery fluid which contains some blood cells. Along the course of the lymph vessels are the *lymph nodes*. These have a defensive function in helping to eliminate foreign matter, including organisms. They also produce some of the white cells involved in the same defences − *lymphocytes*.

The return circulation from the foot to the heart is of particular importance. As the arterial system ends at the extremities, blood returns via the veins from these points. The structures of the foot are highly vascular, and their health is dependent on an adequate supply of blood. The mechanics of the arterial system mean that this is normally achieved. Once the blood has given its food and oxygen to the tissues it flows into a network of veins encircling the pedal bone and covering the lateral cartilages. The return circulation then requires assistance for the uphill flow and compensation for the lowering of the direct pumping force of the heart.

Within the foot, immediately underneath the frog, is the elastic *pedal cushion*. Each time a horse puts his foot to the ground, pressure from the frog exerts a similar pressure on the cushion which is thrust upwards between the lateral cartilages squeezing the blood out of the venous network and into the veins on the way back to the heart. To avoid back-flow the larger veins are provided with valves at intervals.

From all of this it is possible to appreciate that lack of exercise can contribute to faulty limb circulation and, consequently, filled legs.

Two organ systems are closely linked with the circulation, namely *the liver* and *the lungs*.

The Liver

This is one of the most important organs in the body. It is a centre for a great deal of digestive processes as well as being a major organ of detoxification. It also plays a vital part in the body defences. Many of the products of digestion are brought straight to the liver in the hepatic portal system from the bowel.

The major functions of the liver can be listed as follows:

   a. Metabolism of protein, carbohydrate and fat.
   b. Detoxification of harmful substances.
   c. Storage of vitamins.
   d. Destruction of red cells.
   e. Formation of blood proteins.
   f. Secretion of bile.

The liver is also a major producer of lymph.

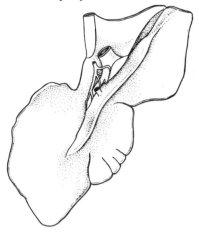

Liver of the horse: posterior view showing the main blood vessels

All this means that the blood leaving the liver is cleaned of toxins and foreign matter which may have entered the circulation from the bowel.

The Lungs

The lungs are part of the respiratory system which is involved in the exchange of gases with the environment. *Oxygen* from inhaled air is bound to molecules within the *red blood cells (RBCs)* and *carbon dioxide* is released into the atmosphere. The exchange occurs at the level of capillaries in the *alveoli* of the lungs. Venous blood is pumped straight to the lungs from the heart and the newly oxygenated blood is returned into the arterial circulation via the heart.

Functions of the Blood

When studying disease it is important that the main functions of the blood be understood, in view of the vital part it plays in maintaining health and combating disease.

Blood is made up of two main parts, liquid and cellular. This is readily seen if a sample is collected into a container holding anti-coagulant — to prevent it from clotting — and allowed to stand. The cells will fall under gravity and the upper fluid — the plasma — is clear and straw coloured. After a short period of time, it is possible to see the red cells at the bottom with a thin coat of white cells on top of them and the plasma overhead. In normal horse blood the column of settled red cells − similar to packed cell volume or PCV − is in the region of 40 per cent. The laboratory test for PCV involves spinning the blood down in a centrifuge to give a more accurate assessment. However, the size of the column in collected samples is a good indicator in gross clinical conditions. It is also possible to note the appearance of bile or blood pigments on occasion; where there is jaundice due to liver disease or excessive breakdown of red blood cells for example.

Serum is the clear fluid which is exuded from clotted blood. It is similar to plasma except for the absence of the factors involved in the clotting process.

Plasma acts as a vehicle for the cells of the blood, and also carries nutritive material in solution, after digestion, from the gut to all parts of the body to aid in tissue growth and repair. It is also the medium through which impurities and waste products are carried back to be neutralised and discharged from the body, via the liver, kidneys, defensive system and skin.

The blood cells are divided into red and white categories; there are also platelets, which are involved in clotting the blood. Arterial blood is bright red in colour, whereas venous blood is darker; this is owing to the different chemical combinations formed by the inhaled and waste gases.

The white cells, known as *leucocytes*, are an integral part of the body defences against disease. They encounter germs and other foreign matter which enter the body and are there to neutralise or destroy them. They also form a critical function in repair of tissues and the healing of wounds. They are listed as follows:

    a. Neutrophils − attack bacterial invaders.
    b. Lymphocytes − involved in immune processes and in fighting viral and bacterial invaders.
    c. Eosinophils − produced in certain allergic conditions, worm infestations.
    d. Monocytes − commonly increased in the blood in some viral diseases.
    e. Basophils − correspond to the mast cells of the tissues.

More will be said about leucocytes later.

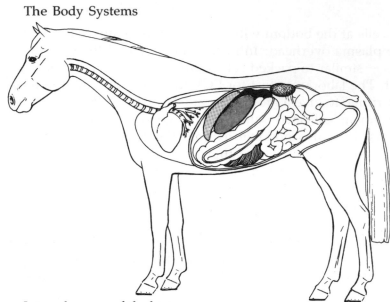

Internal organs of the horse

Digestion

The digestive system consists of the organs directly concerned with the prehension and digestion of food, its passage through the body and the expulsion of waste materials. The gut is a complex hollow structure extending from the lips at one end to the anus at the other. It consists of the *mouth*, housing the *tongue* and *teeth*, the *pharynx* (throat), *oesophagus* (gullet), *stomach*, *small intestine* and *large intestine*.

Associated with these are several structures such as the *salivary glands* and the *pancreas*, which produce secretions vital to the digestive process. The liver is intimately involved in digestion. It plays a critical part in the postabsorption processes involving *protein*, *carbohydrate* and *fat*. While these substances are brought to it directly from the bowel, it is the liver which orchestrates their use within the body. The liver also produces *bile*, which helps the absorption of fat from the bowel, and has other chemical influences on the digestive processes. However, as already stated, it is one of the principle organs of detoxification, and it plays a major role in the body defences.

Food is essential to life, though it is not eaten normally in a form that can be readily used by the body. It has to be digested — broken down — progressively, by the action of various secretions and other physical and biological influences which reduce it to a state in which it can cross the lining of the bowel and enter the vascular system.

Saliva not only lubricates ingested food but it contains enzymes which help in the breakdown of starch. The mechanical effects of chewing are self-evident, but the movement of the jaws also helps the release and mixing of saliva with the ingesta. In the stomach the ingesta meet the enzyme *pepsin*, which is involved in protein digestion, and *hydrochloric acid* which further assists the breakdown of materials. The process is also assisted by the physical massaging effects of the stomach and gut movements, called *peristalsis*. This is a vital factor in moving the food onwards, and it relies greatly on the fibre content of the diet. Further digestive secretions are added by the pancreas, the gall bladder and various glands in the lining of the bowel. While the horse does not have a gall bladder *per se*, it has a continuous outflow of bile from the bile duct to aid digestion.

Add to all this a substantial amount of microbial digestion, particularly in the large bowel, and the complexities of the subject begin to become clear. However, there is an increasing need to understand this subject, because feeding practices are becoming more complex, often challenging the simple nature of the equine digestive system. The result is pressure on the tract leading to indigestion, inflammation of the tissues and even ulceration.

The Ingredients of Food

a. *Carbohydrates* — *glucose* is the characteristic blood sugar, and this is produced from the breakdown of ingested carbohydrates, whether they be from sugars, starches or dietary fibre.

b. *Proteins* constitute about 18 per cent of bodyweight and are essential constituents of all living cells. They are of animal and vegetable origin and are broken down to *amino acids* during the course of digestion.

c. *Fats* are essentially the stored food reserves of the body, though they play a more complex role in metabolism.

d. *Water* — 70 per cent of bodyweight is water.

e. *Vitamins* — essential dietary constituents.

f. *Minerals* — vital to life and required in a constant supply.

g. *Trace elements* — equally important but used in smaller amounts.

The Main Functions of these Components

Carbohydrates are responsible for providing the energy and heat needs of the body.

Protein is vital to growth, maintenance and repair of the animal body.

Fats are involved in energy and heat production. They also form the basis of body reserves used in starvation.

Water is the underlying orchestrator of all living things. Each process and element involved in life exists in a dynamic relationship with it. It is also able to hold large amounts of heat without significantly rising in temperature. This is very significant in the maintenance of body heat within acceptable levels.

Vitamins, *minerals* and *trace elements* are all involved in the various chemical processes which sustain life.

By nature the horse is a muscular, mobile animal dependent to a great extent on his limbs. Horses are used for work of various types, but muscular effort does not require appreciable amounts of protein — the building of muscle does. The energy for this work is derived from the breakdown of carbohydrates which must be readily available from the diet. Carbohydrate is produced within the body by the conversion of fats and, if necessary, protein.

All these essential components must be provided continually, otherwise animals will not be able to develop or perform; body reserves are soon depleted if not replenished.

A certain amount of fibre is essential for stimulation of the bowel. However, where this is too high, the animal is unable to get his energy requirements for work, and the size and bulk of the bowel limit performance. It is for this reason that cereal grains are fed to horses in work. They provide high levels of carbohydrates and protein per unit-weight fed.

By reducing the bulk of hay consumed, the extent of large bowel fermentation is controlled, and the physical bulk of the abdomen is notably smaller. While grass can, under ideal conditions, provide the horse with a great deal of his growth and energy requirements, the problem is that the quality of grass varies in our climate. Horses are, however, raced successfully from the field in parts of the world (with an understanding of the limitations of grass and the added support of controlled hard feeding this requires).

Water is the basis of life. It is required both to maintain body fluid levels and to replace that which is spent under normal use. A great deal is lost through sweating — a part of heat conservation — and other normal body functions, but it is not adequate simply to provide water in replacement when there has been increased demand. Various electrolytes are lost in these processes and they need to be replaced in order to maintain fluid balance. The average horse is said to have a daily water requirement of approximately five gallons.

Nowadays, with the accent on automatic water supplies, it is not always possible to tell what the consumption is, or if, in fact, the animal is drinking at all. Some horses take a mouthful of water with every taste of food, making a track across their box from feed bowl to water trough and back. Individual habits vary as much as with humans, but it is important to know what the individual animal's consumption is so that abnormalities can be quickly detected.

The body demands an adequate intake of minerals for both growing and mature animals. Calcium, phosphorus and magnesium are required for bone formation, and are vital to many of the minute chemical processes of the body. With substances such as sodium chloride — salt — minerals control body fluid levels and keep acidity, or alkalinity, within critical levels. The horse has a high daily requirement of all minerals, and, in the young animal, the needs of growth mean an even greater demand.

Modern nutritional practices are subjecting the horse to a variety of challenges. The animal's tolerance of protein is tested to the full by the use of rations with a greater variety and higher levels of protein in them. This is reflected, however, in an increasing incidence of gastro-enteritis and ulceration of the bowel.

Today's human athletes often reduce protein intake on days immediately prior to a race and increase the volume of carbohydrates eaten. The purpose of this is to facilitate the availability and use of energy. The practice has been tried on horses but with no uniform acceptance of its benefit.

The equine digestive system was designed by nature to fulfil the demands of life in the wild. The horse in such circumstances feeds predominantly on herbivorous material. He covers wide ranges of land, ever alert to the dangers of predators. He has a high energy requirement, and little variety of food.

Under modern methods of management, we move away from this simple system and introduce the animal to increasing varieties of feed. This is a complicating factor of bowel pathology. Its digestion may also prove an added burden for the liver — especially when surplus protein has to be dealt with.

The gut works more efficiently when faced with a simple rather than a complicated diet. For the athlete, digestion should be quick and efficient. Too much variety may lengthen the time food remains in the stomach, predisposing to inflammation of the tissues and improper digestion. The consequence of this is lowered performance.

If excess protein is fed it has to be broken down and stored as fat. The added body weight which results can slow the animal significantly. In conditions where there is disease of the liver, the tolerance of protein is greatly reduced. This is the case after certain virus infections. It can result in marked complications in the muscular system.

It goes without saying that horses being rested need to have their daily food intake reduced. 'Monday Morning Disease', or azoturia, occurred in the past after horses were rested on full rations. The same is equally likely to happen today.

The inevitable conclusion from all this is that the well-being of the animal is in the hands of the feeder. It is important to be able to see if he is holding condition against his work. While this can be helped by weighing, an objective decision has to be made on the basis of appearance. Too fat can be just as great a problem as too light.

Minerals

The principle minerals are as follows: calcium, phosphorus, magnesium, sodium, potassium, chlorine, sulphur, iron, copper, cobalt, iodine, manganese, zinc, molybdenum, selenium and fluorine. Other minerals which occur in tissues are aluminium, arsenic, barium, bromine, cadmium, chromium, silicon and strontium. This list is by no means exhaustive, and only goes to show the intimacy of our relationship with all the elements found in nature.

Calcium and Phosphorus

These minerals act as the major structural elements of skeletal tissue. Most of their body total is found in bones and teeth, which are also the reservoirs for them. During times of added demand − like pregnancy and lactation − these reserves are called upon and mobilised. Both minerals are also vital elements of the blood. They are absorbed into the system in the upper part of the small intestine; a process which is helped by vitamin D. The recommended levels in the diet are 1:1 (Ca:P) for adults and 2:1 for growing or lactating animals. Deficiencies of any of these substances − including the vitamin − can lead to rickets or similar conditions. But deficiencies can occur even when there are adequate amounts in the diet, when there are problems associated with absorption from the bowel.

Magnesium

This mineral is a component of soft tissue and bone − where up to 70 per cent of the body total may be found. It is actively involved in many enzyme systems. Low blood levels can cause serious illness, though this is not common in horses today. The functioning of muscle and nervous tissue depends on a correct balance between calcium and magnesium.

Sodium

This is involved in the regulation of osmotic pressure, acid-base balance and the transmission of nerve impulses.

Potassium

Potassium also plays a part in acid-base balance and osmotic pressure regulation. It is found mainly inside cells, where it plays an important part in muscle contraction. Its absence can lead to muscular paralysis. It has a vital role in certain basic cellular enzyme reactions.

Chlorine

Chlorine is closely related to sodium within the body. It is also associated with hydrogen as part of the acid present in the stomach. It plays a vital part in acid-base balance.

Iodine

Iodine is essential to the formation of thyroid hormones, which are involved in growth.

Sulphur

Sulphur is a constituent of certain amino acids, and is therefore a part of the building processes of some cells.

Fluorine

This is important in the formation of teeth, and normally present in bones as well.

Selenium

Selenium is a part of certain enzymes. It is tied in with vitamin E, and deficiencies relate to the condition known as white muscle disease in foals. Selenium is known to be deficient in certain areas.

Molybdenum

This mineral is involved in a number of enzyme systems. It is known that excessive liming of land can cause a deficiency of molybdenum.

Iron

Iron is a part of the haemoglobin molecule responsible for the transport of oxygen in the blood. It is also part of the myoglobin molecule of muscle, and contained in certain enzymes.

Copper

A great deal of body copper is contained in the liver, where it plays an active role in enzyme systems. It interplays with dietary molybdenum, and is also actively involved in the early formation of red blood cells.

Cobalt

Cobalt is a component of vitamin B12.

Zinc

Zinc is involved in enzyme systems, one of the functions of which is to aid carbon dioxide transport in the blood and its release in the lungs.

Manganese

Manganese is a constituent of enzyme systems involved in protein and fat metabolism.

Vitamins

Vitamins are unrelated organic compounds which play an active role in metabolism. Some are contained in ingested food while others are synthesised in the animal body from constituents which arrive in food. Organisms involved in digestion may play a part in this, for example, vitamin B12, known as the 'animal protein factor', is not available from vegetable sources It can, however, be synthesised in the bowel by organisms.

Vitamin A

This vitamin is important for bone formation and vision. It plays a part in maintaining the health of cells which line body structures and, therefore, helps with disease resistance. It is essential for normal development of the young animal, and for reproduction. The vitamin is formed in the body from precursors which are available from grass and vegetables such as carrots. Feeding too much can cause toxicity. Large amounts of the precursor are lost in the curing and storage of hay.

Vitamin D

Vitamin D facilitates the absorption of calcium and phosphorus from the intestine and assists them in the formation of bone. It is found in hay, and is synthesised in the skin on exposure to sunlight. Fish oils are a rich source. Absence of sunlight may cause a deficiency.

Vitamin E

Vitamin E is a factor in reproduction, but it also plays a major part in the integrity of the muscular system. It is inter-related with selenium, with which it helps to prevent muscular dystrophy. Cereal grains, green plants and hay are good sources.

Vitamin K

This vitamin is important to the clotting mechanism of blood. It is generally synthesised in the intestine of animals. Hay and pasture are rich sources.

B Vitamins

Vitamin B1 (Thiamine) This is vital to cell metabolism. Brewer's yeast is a very good source, as are cereal grains and hay.

Riboflavin is involved with energy metabolism. It is found widely in nature.

Niacin is involved with glucose metabolism. Brewer's yeast is a good source.

Vitamin B6 (pyridoxine) is important to protein metabolism. It is widely available in nature and deficiencies are unlikely under normal dietary conditions.

Pantothenic acid is actively involved with metabolism. It is found widely in nature.

Vitamin B12 This is also known as the anti-pernicious-anaemia factor, describing the part it plays in blood metabolism. It is a vitamin not contained in any vegetable source and is synthesised by organisms in the gut of the horse. However, although deficiencies are said to be unlikely in practice, the supplementation of this vitamin to horses is often seen to have a significant beneficial effect.

Folic acid is concerned with red-cell formation and is commonly added to equine feed supplements.

Biotin is important to carbon dioxide fixation and in metabolism. It is universally available.

Choline

Choline is involved in metabolism and is universally available.

Vitamin C

Vitamin C is important to the maintenance of a healthy epithelium. Fresh fruits are a good source, as are greens including grass. The horse can synthesise it in the liver.

As has already been said, grass can provide all the necessary ingredients of a balanced diet, but its bulk is one of the problems for working horses. This problem is partly solved by drying, but in the process vitamin values are reduced. These are lowered further by bad harvesting because vitamins are affected adversely by excessive heat and fermentation as well as by too much sun. Kiln drying of grain can also destroy it.

Where a diet contains a good class hay (cut young so that the seed is not lost) oats, bran and carrots, an ample supply of most of the vitamins will be present. Reputable feed compounders are careful that their products cater for the same need anyway. However there are innumerable feed supplements available as well.

For young, growing animals the need for a balanced intake of essential vitamins and minerals cannot be overstressed. Deficiencies will occur when there is any shortage, and the most common of these are ricket-type conditions associated with bone development. This must not be confused with enlargements of the epiphyseal plates in foals due to hard ground — most noticeable on fetlock joints. In this case, the animal will grow into the leg and the enlargements will disappear in time. However it is very important in both situations to assess the diet and ensure there is no imbalance of calcium and phosphorus, and adequate vitamins A, D and E.

Foals fed on oats and bran need a balanced intake of these same substances. Bran is a rich source of phosphorus and fed alone can cause disease in horses of any age. Where foals are fed on grain it is necessary to ensure vitamins and minerals are being provided.

Before leaving this subject, it should be mentioned that excessive supplies of vitamins are unnecessary and may be harmful. Specific symptoms result from vitamin deficiencies, and from excesses. Foals kept in dark stables may be short of vitamin D (the sunshine vitamin), but feeding excessive amounts of the same vitamin causes toxicity.

All of the B-vitamin complex is commonly available from normal food sources, or are synthesised in the gut of the horse by micro-organisms. However deficiencies may occur where there is added demand — as with the racehorse — so it is important that supplements are available where needed.

Excretion

Waste is a normal by-product of metabolism. The body exists in a dynamic state where there are chemical reactions going on at all times. The exhalation of carbon dioxide is a simple indication of this process. There are waste products of digestion as well as of many other processes within the body. Bile is a means of getting rid of the waste pigments of blood breakdown, and the bile pigments colour the faeces. The kidney is the pathway for the elimination of urea, which is a by-product of protein metabolism.

It is vital to life that this process of cleansing the body of waste is functional and ongoing. Ill health is the inevitable outcome of any failure. If the kidneys fail there is a condition called uraemia, which is very toxic. Constipation also has a toxic effect and unless relieved the animal will suffer; it can induce colic and death.

It must also be understood that there are many stages of abnormality which need to be observed. A horse may not be constipated but the faeces may have adopted an abnormal consistency, colour or smell. These are all signs of inner influences of one kind or another and need to be watched and logged. They provide information which is vital in any clinical examination.

Skin

The skin plays a part, with the kidneys, in the control of fluid balance and heat control. If sweating is restricted the kidneys will increase their output: in cold weather more urine is passed, and vice versa. The primary functions of the skin are:

    a. To mechanically protect the body.
    b. To keep out toxic agents.
    c. To prevent excess water loss.
    d. Protection against irradiation.
    e. Heat control.
    f. Sensation — all sensations are subject to nerves which penetrate the skin.

g. Secretion of sweat and sebum.

h. Formation of vitamin D.

The skin is able to absorb substances from outside which are fat or water soluble.

Sweat

This is one of the most dilute body fluids and its function is to control heat within the body. The process of sweating is designed to remove from the system excess heat produced through exercise, or infection. This happens by general irradiation from the body surface and by evaporation of sweat which cools the skin generally. The internal body temperature is kept within the narrow limits compatible with life — about 101 °F (37–38 °C)   at the expense of the body fluids. When there is an increased activity of the body and greater heat formed within, blood vessels of the skin surface expand to radiate heat and stimulate the sweat glands to produce perceptible amounts of sweat. In cold weather these blood vessels contract, reducing the circulation of the skin and therefore the amount of blood which is exposed to the cooling action of the air outside; the sweat glands show a significant reduction in output.

The expulsion of sweat involves the contraction of muscle cells surrounding the ducts, or pores, of sweat glands. These act in response to central stimulation and to chemical substances present in the circulating blood. As we all know, many horses sweat if they are worried, e.g. when travelling, which has nothing to do with heat regulation.

Sweat does not play a significant part in body waste excretion.

With infection, an increase of temperature is a specific defensive response to the presence of organisms. The temperature rise is an action of the body designed to eliminate the intruder. Sweating may well occur in this situation, though it is by no means inevitable. In the past drugs have been used to combat infection because of their ability to promote sweating, thereby reducing body heat. However, this type of drug is not commonly used on the horse today; antibiotics have a more specific effect on infection.

Sweating is a natural side-effect of exercise. It is the body's way of controlling the extra heat produced by increased energy use.

Sebum

This is an oily, wax-like substance secreted by glands which are found all over the skin. The function of the secretion is to coat and protect the hair from drying out, overwetting and other physical damage. It makes the coat shiny and sleek, provides a form of insulation, and is part of the protective mechanism of the skin.

Grooming is extremely important for the horse as a means of keeping the skin clean and the sweat pores in a healthy condition.

Clothing is necessary to retain body heat when the natural coat has been clipped off. It is an essential addendum to this that the environment in which the horse is stabled is warm and supports this purpose of retaining body heat.

The Kidneys

The kidneys are two in number and are situated to either side of the midline in the lumbar region of the back, in front of the pelvis.

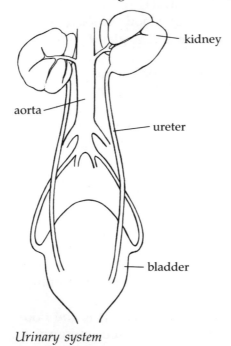

Urinary system

Their functions are mainly excretory, and are:

    a. Control of water balance.
    b. Elimination of waste products of protein metabolism.
    c. Control of blood acid-base balance.
    d. Elimination of other compounds — certain drugs are excreted
       by the kidneys.

Urine

The urine of the horse is thick or syrupy in consistency because of a high mucus content. It is normally turbid when passed because of calcium carbonate crystals suspended in it.

The Nervous System

The *brain* and *spinal cord* form the *central nervous system* which is a very complicated structure, and we shall deal with its functions only (not its anatomy) as these have a great bearing on health and disease.

Most movement, function and sensation occurs through the sending of a message from the central nervous system and its interpretation by the organ receiving it. This is not the case with certain *reflexes*, which respond locally.

Every part of the body is supplied with nerves from the brain or spinal cord, and should this nerve supply be cut off the part ceases to function. In extreme illness, nerve impulses may be slowed down and weak.

To simplify understanding of this subject, nerves are divided into:

    a. *Motor nerves* regulating movement.
    b. *Sensory nerves* registering sensation.
    c. *Autonomic nerves* are another system of nerves acting on the
       bowel and blood, including the heart. These are outside vol-
       untary control and need not be discussed here.

Two examples of different types of body function will suffice to demonstrate how the nervous system works.

Example 1   When a pin or other sharp object is applied to the skin, an animal will try to withdraw from the offending impulse.

The pin touches a nerve-ending in the skin of the lower leg, for example, and the pain impulse is transferred by the sensory nerve to the spinal cord. On arrival the impulse is connected with a motor impulse which is passed out from the spinal cord, down the motor nerves to the muscles of the forearm and the foot is snatched from the ground. This is a purely reflex action without any assistance or control from the brain.

Meanwhile the brain has received the pain sensation and an impulse goes out to the muscles of the limbs, causing the whole body to be moved away from the offending impulse. The horse may also kick out to defend himself. The first part of the response was not voluntary, the second was.

Example 2   A sudden movement of an object towards an eye causing the closing of the eyelids as a protection for the eyeball.

The nerves of sight register the danger and carry the impulse to the brain, from which emanate impulses to the retractor muscles of the eyeball causing it to be pulled back into its socket and so allowing the *nictitating membrane* (haw) to flick across the eye. At the same time impulses pass to the muscles controlling the *eyelids*, causing them to contract and pull the eyelids over the *eyeball*.

These two examples concern impulses via nerves controlling voluntary movement. It is simple to see the difference between reflex responses in which the nervous system takes control and voluntary responses which are within the control of the will. The immediate response to a stimulus may be outside voluntary control − reflex − while the decision to kick is a matter of choice.

The smell or sight of food will stimulate the secretion of saliva. Similarly contact of food with the walls of the bowel causes movement and the secretion of other substances. Neither of these acts is voluntary.

Within the skin atmospheric temperature will influence the state of contraction or dilatation of blood vessels and the output of the sweat glands.

With the knowledge that all functions can be effected only by stimulation from a nerve impulse and that the latter will be weak in certain situations, such as disease, dietary deficiencies, fatigue, etc., good horsemastership and stable management must be directed towards the elimination of these problems. *Fatigue* occurs when the energy required for immediate further exercise is exhausted. It is a complex condition which relates not only to energy but water and electrolyte balance as well. It is inevitably more common when an animal is unfit. The whole process of training is designed to prepare the body for greater amounts of work. This includes the development of the heart and lung circulations as well as the changes which occur in muscle to allow for the added effort required.

Fatigue may well occur when the horse is subjected to too much work. It is reversed by rest, feed and proper electrolyte supplementation. It should be understood that absorption is a vital factor in electrolyte levels in the blood. There can be adequate quantities in the food and the animal may be *dehydrated* because of faulty absorption. There are many electrolyte formulae available on the market, though they are not all equally effective.

Electrolytes play a part in holding water in solution in the blood. In their absence the animal is dehydrated, because of relative water shortage in the blood system. The PCV rises and the blood does not circulate so readily because it thickens. It is easy to understand that the heart would have greater difficulty in pumping it around in that state.

Some horses break out after hard work, producing what is often referred to as a 'cold sweat' when back in the stable. They may be dried off, but will break out again shortly. This condition is an expression of eletrolyte imbalance and is effectively treated by ensuring that their levels are restored to normal. Electrolytes may be given either in the drinking water or food. They may be given by drench or stomach tube, or, alternatively, given in drip form intravenously when the condition warrants it.

3   Conformation

Because bad conformation predisposes to injury or disease the subject warrants serious consideration.

Over the years, breeding has gravitated towards the production of certain ideals associated with speed, strength, temperament, movement, etc. This, naturally, has related to the type of use for which the particular horse was intended. Judges tend very often to have their own idea of what is best, but there are people in existence whose ability to judge a horse for a specific purpose has marked them as masters of the art. Very often even they cannot explain what it is that attracts them. It may be instinctive, but it is a talent which is very hard to come by without learning and experience.

Head

A good head should be of a size proportionate to the horse; a head that is too big tends to unbalance the animal. The muzzle should be well defined with large but not dilated nostrils and the straight faceline should be wide and flat between the eyes. A good width should exist between the branches of the lower jaw. Narrow space restricts the movement of the throat and is thought to be associated with unsoundness of wind. The lips cover the upper and lower incisor teeth which should meet at the tables. If the lower teeth are behind the upper teeth (parrot mouth) the animal may not be able to graze properly, especially on short keep. This fault is considered to be hereditary and is not accepted in stallions used for breeding purposes in most countries.

Eyes

The eyes should be large, prominent and clear with uniformly curved lids.

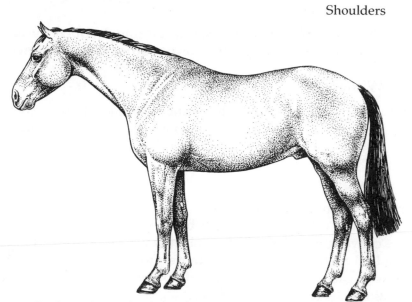

Conformation: a head that is too big tends to unbalance the animal

Ears

Ears should be well placed and alert. Drooping ears have been considered to be a sign of sluggishness, though some very good families of horses have carried this characteristic through their better members. Long ears are said to be associated with speed!

Neck

This should be straight and not too heavy since the carriage of the head is largely dependent on the shape of the neck. A ewe neck may indicate uncertain temperament. The angle at which the head is set on the neck is also important; if too acute it may restrict the larynx and, thus, the breathing.

Shoulders

There should be a good slope from the point of the shoulder to the withers; the greater the slope (within reason) the more efficient the shock-absorber effect to the forelimbs. On the contrary, if the shoulder is too upright, the stride is short and choppy. The pasterns will generally follow the pattern of the horse's shoulders, and the animal may stand over (i.e. the feet are behind a perpendicular line dropped through the point of the shoulder to the ground) or be too straight in front.

Withers

Well defined and pronounced, the withers should slope away gently from top to bottom. Good withers help a correctly fitting saddle to stay in place, but flat withers may allow a saddle to slip forward.

Back

A short back is generally stronger. A long back that dips is likely to lead to eventual weakness. A roach back is the opposite to a dipped back (i.e. convex) and may lead to problems with the fitting of a saddle.

A long-backed horse stands over more ground and covers a greater distance with each stride. Short-backed horses may be faster — this is a conformational feature of the sprinter.

Loins and Hindquarters

The loin is the weakest part of the back because it has the least structural support. Ideally the loins should, therefore, be short and well muscled. The muscle transmits the propulsive power to the trunk. The back is subjected to considerable force when the horse is jumping and can be the cause of a particular type of lameness.

The hindquarters should be strong, muscular and well developed. There should be a good length from hip to hock, and well-muscled second thighs (gaskins), though these too vary with type. In many good jumpers the quarters fall away from the spine, giving them a pointed appearance on top. This 'point' is called a 'jumping bump'. On the other hand, sprinters usually have well-rounded and powerful quarters which give them the speed required to race the shorter distances.

Girth and Ribs

Long and well-sprung ribs provide a large space in which to house the heart and lungs which are essential organs for the competing athlete. With a horse with good conformation, the measurement around the girth is greater than the height.

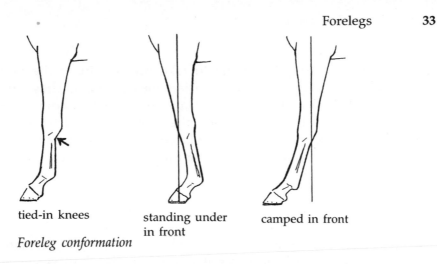

tied-in knees   standing under   camped in front
in front

Foreleg conformation

Forelegs

The expression 'both forelegs coming out of the same hole', although
an exaggeration, aptly describes a narrow-chested horse and signifies a
restricted chest cavity. Further, if the forelegs are closer together, they
are more likely to cause brushing. The elbows should be clearly defined
and set out from the body.

Forearms

A weak forearm denotes lack of muscle and can also indicate weakness
of the related tendons.

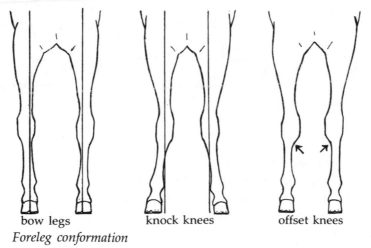

bow legs   knock knees   offset knees

Foreleg conformation

Knees

These should be broad and flat to take the weight of the body. The knees, if not strong, are prone to lameness, and, if they are out of proportion to the body, will not stand the strain. Looking from the front, the bone of the forearm and the cannon should be in a straight line with the knee, which must be placed centrally between them. If the line of these three entities is not continuous, an uneven strain will be placed on the knee.

Over at the Knee

This is the term given to the foreleg when the knee sits permanently in a position forward of the straight line when the limb is viewed from the side. It may be the result of contracted tendons or may be conformational. The tendons in such a limb are under less strain, and many good judges discount the fault if the animal has ability.

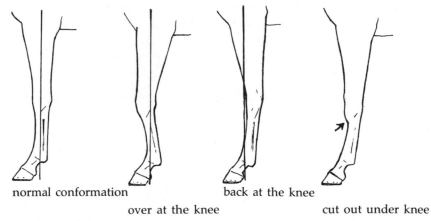

normal conformation   back at the knee

over at the knee   cut out under knee

Foreleg conformation

Back at the Knee

This term is applied to a horse whose foreleg shows a slightly concave profile when viewed from the side. The knee joint sits behind the straight line. It is a bad fault indicating weakness of the tendons and a knee joint which is subjected to a crunching action at the point of concussion.

Cannon Bone

This bone should be short and strong with clearly defined tendons behind it. 'Bone' is a term meant to convey the measurement of the cannon region, in circumference, beneath the knee. This measurement incorporates both the bone and the tendons. The term 'a good span' means that the tendons are well developed, as well as the bone.

The term 'tied in below the knee' describes a fault where the measurement below the knee is less than the measurement further down the leg, and, as a result, the bone and tendon are weak. As a rough guide a good weight-carrying horse should have between eight and nine inches of bone.

Fetlocks

The fetlock rests between the cannon bone and the pastern. It includes two proximal sesamoid bones at the back of the leg. The joint should be clear of swellings, well rounded, and appear neither too big nor too small for the limb.

Pasterns

A good pastern is set at a gentle angle; the more sloping the pastern, the greater the strain on the suspensory ligament and tendons, thus predisposing both to injury, but if the pastern is upright, concussion is not buffered but registered directly on the joints. The angle of the foreleg pasterns should approximate 45–50 degrees to the ground, and the angle of the hind leg pastern should be 50–55 degrees. This line should run straight down the foot to the ground and should break neither forward nor backward at the coronet.

Feet

The hoof should be deep and wide between the heels; this is called an 'open foot'. Narrow, boxy feet restrict the physiological function of the sensitive structures and so predispose to disease. The frog should be well developed with a shallow median depression.

Occasionally a horse may have odd-sized feet, but this is not necessarily detrimental.

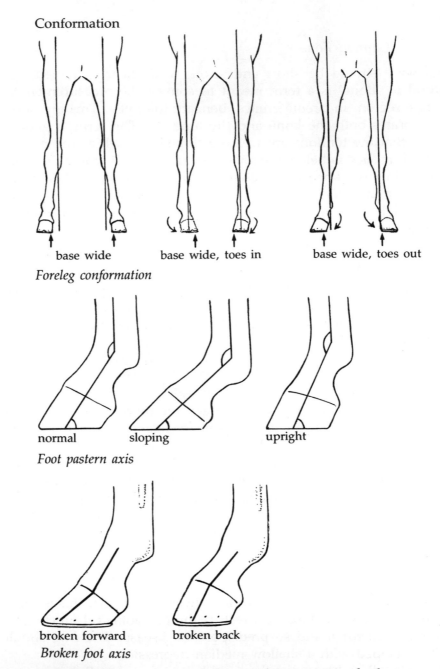

base wide   base wide, toes in   base wide, toes out

Foreleg conformation

normal   sloping   upright

Foot pastern axis

broken forward   broken back

Broken foot axis

The horn should have a level surface without any marked grooves or rings and no signs of contraction of the quarters.

The colour of the horn has a certain significance, unpigmented horn being fundamentally weaker.

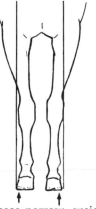 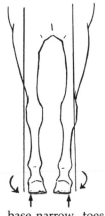 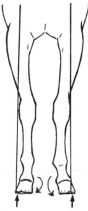

base narrow, weight on outside of foot   base narrow, toes in   base narrow, toes out

Foreleg conformation

Turned-in Toes

This is not good conformation as it leads to stumbling and also places a strain on the structures of the leg.

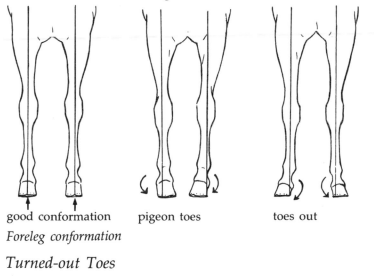

good conformation   pigeon toes   toes out

Foreleg conformation

Turned-out Toes

This fault may cause brushing and also places a strain on leg structures.

Hind Legs

The *thighs* should be long and well muscled. There should not be a lot of daylight between them when viewed from behind. The second thigh, or gaskin, should be strong, because the muscles which activate the hock and foot originate in this area.

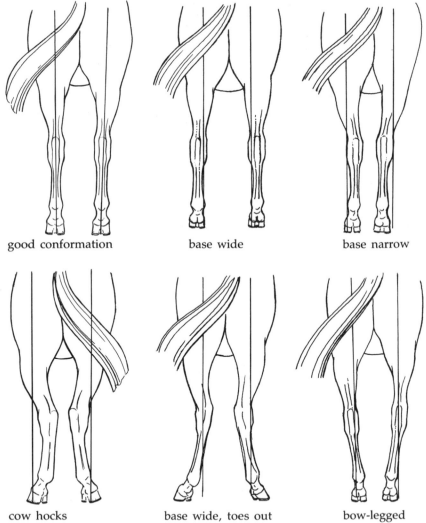

| good conformation | base wide | base narrow |
| cow hocks | base wide, toes out | bow-legged |

Hind leg conformation

Hocks

These should be strong and well constructed when viewed from the side. If they turn inwards when viewed from the back — cow hocks — it is a sign of weakness.

If the point of the hock is too well defined, giving the impression that the joint is over-flexed, greater strain falls on the point of curb (at the lower end of the back of the hock). These hocks are known as sickle hocks.

A straight hock, the reverse of the former, is often a strong joint, though the Achilles tendon inserted into the point of it is more likely to give trouble. Nevertheless, several celebrated lines of Thoroughbred horses, such as the St. Simon stock, had very straight hocks and had no problems despite vigorous training.

Cannons, Fetlocks, Pasterns and Feet

In each case the conformation points are the same as those of the forelegs.

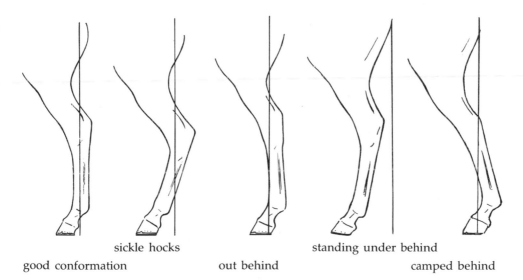

good conformation   sickle hocks   out behind   standing under behind   camped behind

Hind leg conformation

4   Description

From many points of view it is useful to know how to describe a horse, either when advertising for sale or during a discussion. Unless accepted procedures are adopted an accurate picture will not be drawn. Horses are described according to breeding and useage.

Thoroughbred

A Thoroughbred is a horse which is entitled to be recorded in the General Stud Book kept by Weatherbys. For a horse to be eligible for registration, it must be possible to trace all his lines of pedigree to horses registered before 1st January, 1980 in the *General Stud Book*. Alternatively, the horse may have been included in any of a list of stud books as agreed by the International Stud Book Committee from time to time.

In certain circumstances non-thoroughbreds can be promoted to Thoroughbred, providing it can be proved that in their pedigree they have eight consecutively recorded crosses with Thoroughbreds (as defined above). It must also be shown that certain performance criteria are met in their pedigrees.

Most Thoroughbreds are registered when foals in the first four months of life. To encourage early registration, fees are lower at this time. The procedure involves proper identification, including blood typing.

As adults, these horses are registered by name for racing, and this may be done at any time from the yearling stage onwards. The Jockey Club are not in favour of changing names once registered. When registration is complete, a passport is issued. This may include such information as the horse's name, the current owner, trainer, identifying markings, breeding, and record of vaccinations. It will also record if a mare or stallion has retired from racing to stud.

In general, the majority of foal markings will have been taken by the end of July in the year of foaling, together with blood samples. The blood is placed into containers, supplied by Weatherbys, and submitted to the Animal Health Trust at Newmarket. Here the blood type is checked against those of sire and dam to confirm parentage. Providing this test raises no queries, and after the foal registration formalities have been completed, the passport is issued and should accompany the horse from then on. This ensures that his identity can be checked whenever necessary.

Marking Forms

When filling in marking forms, the details and marking of all horses should be written using the terms, colours etc. as described in the following sections.

Colour

Black, brown, bay, bay brown, chestnut, grey and roan are the colours for Thoroughbred horses. The colour roan is seldom a true colour in Thoroughbreds, as there is often a mixture of grey and chestnut, or white hairs running through the body coats of chestnuts and bays.

Sometimes, at foal stage, colours are not very well defined. Double colour descriptions such as 'chestnut or grey' are accepted at this time. Where there is doubt about a foal's true colour, the muzzle and eyelids are examined for further guidance.

For non-thoroughbreds additional colours given are piebald, skewbald, cream, yellow or blue dun, and blue, bay, red, strawberry or chestnut roan. Odd-coloured defines a situation where there are more than two colours in the body coat. There is also palomino, which is a distinct gold colour combined with white mane and tail; and Appaloosa, which is not a defined colour but a body pattern of colours as defined by the breed society.

Sex

Colt, filly, gelding, horse or mare.

NC1 NAMING FORM

(Effective under the Rules of Racing)

REGISTRATION FEE

(INCLUDING VAT)
(Fees valid until 31/12/88)
Yearlings £13.80
2 and 3 year olds £28.75
4 year olds and up £115.00
Change of name £23.00

☐ Tick if VAT invoice required
(VAT registered persons only)
☐ I enclose cheque £ ....
☐ Please charge my Weatherby account

Account number ☐☐☐☐☐☐☐

FOR OFFICE USE ONLY

Please tick if a passport is required: RACING ☐ STUD ☐

I have enclosed the Foal Identity and Vaccination Certificate for this horse or if foreign bred, identity documents as issued by the Turf Authority concerned ☐

COLOUR	SEX	YEAR FOALED 19 ....

Registered Name of Dam		Registered Name of Sire
		Sire of Dam

NAME OF BREEDER		COUNTRY OF FOALING

USE BLOCK LETTERS

Proposed Names in order of preference
(Please give four choices)

1. .... 3. ....

2. .... 4. ....

For the rules governing availability of names, refer to Rules of Racing, Appendix E

If the horse was foaled prior to 1974 and cannot be accepted for inclusion in the General Stud Book the pedigree of the dam must be entered here.

INSTRUCTIONS

A name cannot be registered for a horse before it is a yearling unless it was foaled elsewhere than in Great Britain, Ireland or the Channel Islands, or is outside these countries at the date of registration.

If the horse was foaled in 1974 or after it must have been accepted for inclusion in the General Stud Book or the Register of Non-Thoroughbred Mares as the produce of a registered sire and dam in order for it to be named.

If the horse is owned in partnership the names of all the partners should be stated. The signature of one will be sufficient.

No confirmation of this registration, other than publication in the Racing Calendar, will be given unless a stamped addressed envelope is enclosed.

Names of well-known persons or names which would act as an advertisement for a Company or product may not be accepted without written authorisation from the person or body concerned.

The Stewards of the Jockey Club have instructed that a Naming Form must be completed in respect of any Foreign-bred horse arriving in training in this country. The Racing Passport, if available, should also be submitted and will be returned after any necessary amendments have been made to the markings.

The Stewards of the Jockey Club may exercise their powers under Rule 1(vii) and (viii) and Rule 31(xii) to cancel a registration of a name or to refuse to allow a horse duly entered to run in any race, inter alia, if at any time a blood test does not confirm the pedigree stated.

I hereby certify that, after due enquiry from previous owners, the above particulars are all that I have been able to ascertain in order to establish the identity and antecedents of the horse described overleaf, and I request that the name now claimed may be registered in accordance with the Rules of Racing.

Name of Owner (in block letters) ....
Please state title (Mr., Mrs., or Miss)

Address of Owner
and trainer if
applicable ....

Telephone number ....

Signature of Owner or Agent ....

Date ....

FOR OFFICE USE ONLY

CAL	T.I.

JOCKEY CLUB RACING CALENDAR OFFICE, WEATHERBYS, SANDERS ROAD, WELLINGBOROUGH, NORTHAMPTONSHIRE, NN8 4BX

Marking form – front (by permission of Weatherbys of Wellingborough)

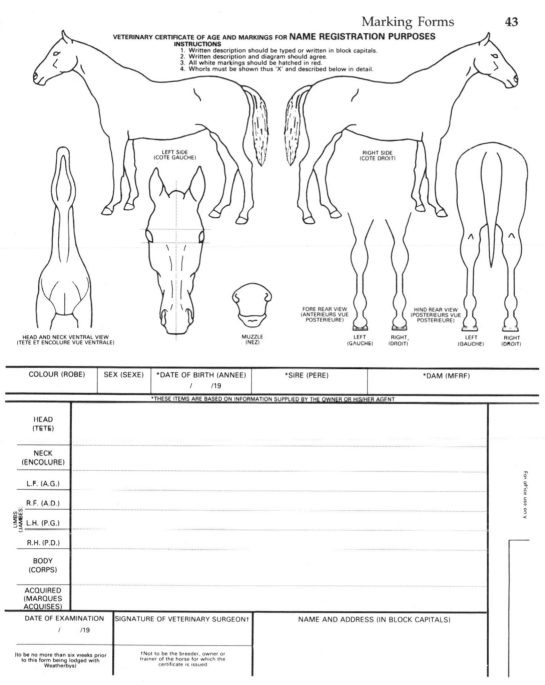

VETERINARY CERTIFICATE OF AGE AND MARKINGS FOR NAME REGISTRATION PURPOSES

INSTRUCTIONS
1. Written description should be typed or written in block capitals.
2. Written description and diagram should agree.
3. All white markings should be hatched in red.
4. Whorls must be shown thus 'X' and described below in detail.

LEFT SIDE (COTE GAUCHE)

RIGHT SIDE (COTE DROIT)

HEAD AND NECK VENTRAL VIEW (TETE ET ENCOLURE VUE VENTRALE)

MUZZLE (NEZ)

FORE REAR VIEW (ANTERIEURS VUE POSTERIEURE)

HIND REAR VIEW (POSTERIEURS VUE POSTERIEURE)

LEFT (GAUCHE) RIGHT (DROIT) LEFT (GAUCHE) RIGHT (DROIT)

COLOUR (ROBE)	SEX (SEXE)	*DATE OF BIRTH (ANNEE) / /19	*SIRE (PERE)	*DAM (MERE)

*THESE ITEMS ARE BASED ON INFORMATION SUPPLIED BY THE OWNER OR HIS/HER AGENT

HEAD (TETE)	
NECK (ENCOLURE)	
L.F. (A.G.)	
R.F. (A.D.)	
L.H. (P.G.)	
R.H. (P.D.)	
BODY (CORPS)	
ACQUIRED (MARQUES ACQUISES)	

LIMBS (JAMBES)

For office use only

DATE OF EXAMINATION / /19	SIGNATURE OF VETERINARY SURGEON†	NAME AND ADDRESS (IN BLOCK CAPITALS)
(to be no more than six weeks prior to this form being lodged with Weatherbys)	†Not to be the breeder, owner or trainer of the horse for which the certificate is issued	

Marking form — back

Date of Birth

This is as supplied by the owner or breeder. A Thoroughbred foal becomes a yearling on the 1st of January of the year after his birth — even when born in the previous December.

Pedigree

The names of both parents, including country code suffixes of sire and dam are entered on the marking form. The suffixes only apply in the case of foreign-bred animals, e.g. FR for France, IRE for Ireland, USA for the United States of America, etc.

Markings

These are drawn on the marking form and described in writing. White markings are now indicated by hatching (parallel or crossed lines), and flesh marks are shaded on the drawing. Official marking forms require at least five identifying marks to be noted.

Head

The shape, size and position of any star, stripe, blaze, white face, snip, white muzzle or lip markings are described. The position of all whorls is recorded and described in perspective, relating to other markings and anatomical landmarks.

Neck

The position of all whorls is described, including those on the crest and on the underside of the neck. A ventral view (front, underside of the body) is provided for whorls and other markings that occur there. With Thoroughbreds, if there are no crest whorls, this must be stated.

Limbs

All markings, including hoof markings and whorls are shown. The hoof may be described as pigmented, unpigmented or partly pigmented.

Body

All markings and their position are described. Different coloured hairs, especially in mane and tail, are recorded, and all whorls shown and described. Specific *spots*, *patches*, *zebra marks* and *lists* are shown and recorded in writing.

Mane and Tail

The presence of differently coloured hairs in the mane and tail are specified.

Acquired Marks

All permanent acquired marks such as saddle marks, firing marks, surgical scars and tattoos are shown.

Congenital Marks

Wall eyes, prophet's thumb marks, lop ears, a parrot mouth and other dental irregularities are recorded.

As will be appreciated, the presence and position of whorls is critical for animals with no other identifying marks.

There is a booklet available on the subject of marking horses issued by the Royal College of Veterinary Surgeons.

Hunter

Type for showing purposes:

Heavyweight —	capable of carrying 89 kg (14 st.) or over.
Middleweight —	capable of carrying between 79.5 kg (12 st. 7 lb.) and 89 kg (14 st.)
Lightweight —	capable of carrying up to 79.5 kg (12 st. 7 lb.)
Working hunter —	light — up to 82.7 kg (13 st.)
	heavy — over 82.7 kg (13 st.)
Small hunter	
Ladies hunter	

Hunter Breeding

There are many varieties of hunter, e.g. a *half-bred* — by a Thoroughbred horse out of a hunter mare. This animal will have to show the quality of the Thoroughbred. It may also be by a non-thoroughbred horse out of a Thoroughbred mare, where the offspring will be expected to show particular qualities of the sire. The cross may be with a light draught, such as the *Irish Draught*, or with a heavier type, such as the *Hanoverian*. The purpose of breeding in this way is to bring some new qualities to the offspring, a process which may be followed through a number of generations. Often the best quality hunters are three or four moves away from the original cross.

Less well-bred hunters are described accordingly, by weight-carrying capacity, shape, and usage.

Point-to-pointers

Point-to-pointers are mostly Thoroughbred, although any animal registered in Weatherbys' Non-Thoroughbred Register is eligible to race in point-to-points and under Jockey Club rules.

Three-day-eventers

These horses are very often Thoroughbred, but the description must fit the ability and scope of the animal to compete at the level for which it is being sold. This goes for any description being given about a horse put up for sale, and the law today does not allow for misrepresentation.

Show-jumpers

Show-jumpers are all sizes, shapes, breeds and types; the only stipulation being, therefore, that they are suitable for the purpose. However, if the horse is a Thoroughbred, half-bred, Arab, Connemara, etc., this information is of particular interest to the buyer and should be stated.

Team Chasers

These horses are as varied in type as the last category, but must be able to compete at the level for which they are sold. In other words, descriptions have to be accurate and a novice cannot be presented as a mature or experienced animal. If he does not fit the description a horse would be returnable in law.

Description of Type and Usage

Horses and ponies described as ready for *driving* must have been broken to harness and, again, fit the purpose for which they are designated.

Hack

The present day hack is a lightweight, quality animal, perhaps even in the *Stud Book*, with good action and measuring about 15–15.3 hh.

Cob

The cob may be a heavyweight or lightweight animal, thick-set and close-coupled. In the past it referred to a short-tailed animal but docking is now illegal.

Child's Pony

This may be of any breed, which should be stated, for example, *Welsh* (with grade recorded), *Shetland*, *Dartmoor*, *Exmoor*, *Connemara*, etc. Height, which has to be exact, is critical in the sale of ponies, especially because the purchaser will wish the pony to suit a child of a particular size and age, and may want to compete in classes for those under the pony's given height.

Other Description Factors

In addition to the aforementioned, there is no harm in describing other factors relating to the animal.

Height

Height is measured in hands (a hand being four inches), and must be accurate and sustainable. In other words, if you advertise your horse as measuring 15′ 2″hh, the animal would, under most conditions of sale, be returnable unless the advertised height was very close to the realistic height. To an extent purchasers are expected to satisfy themselves regarding this, but a little leniency would be allowed, except with ponies which fall under the scope of the Joint Measurement Scheme, and which will have current certificates of height which are binding.

Mouth

Good, light, fussy, hard, one-sided; there are many types of mouth, and while you may not wish to describe an animal as a hard puller, or having any special defect, the purchaser is entitled to know, and the animal may well be returnable if the description is inaccurate. It is always best to be honest.

When buying a horse, remember that many people are selling animals because they have a flaw. It is, therefore, wise to have advice on purchasing, and to obtain warranties as to soundness, age, temperament, vices, etc. A veterinary examination of soundness is usually very worthwhile. It is also worth asking the vendor to guarantee that the animal is not on any drugs at the time of examination.

Manners

Manners are described as good, unreliable or uncertain, or perhaps, hot. It is worth remembering that a child injured on a pony which was patently temperamentally unsuitable, may have a claim against the vendor if it is possible to prove that the vendor was aware of the fact before selling.

Movement

Free, good, poor, sluggish or fast.

Action

Straight, choppy, toe-in or toe-out. Inevitably these descriptions are excluded if not in the animal's favour. The purchaser should be in a position to judge them anyway.

Ride

Good, moderate, staying (maybe suitable for endurance riding).

In Traffic

Will pass anything, safe; nervous of heavy vehicles, unsuitable.

Age

The age of older horses is quite accurately gauged by dentition and this is described in detail in the next chapter.

5 Dentition

The ageing of horses is a subject which can cause considerable difference of opinion. The argument concerns the teeth and the part they play in estimating age. Like all other animals, the horse has two sets of teeth during his life, the first known as temporary or milk teeth, which are replaced by permanent teeth as the animal matures.

According to their position in the jaw bones, the teeth are classified as follows.

a. *Incisor teeth* − There are six incisors in both lower and upper jaws. The wearing surface has a depression in the centre of each tooth, called the infundibulum, or mark, which disappears gradually with age. The shape of the incisors varies being oval at the top and gradually tapering to triangular at the root. Their purpose is cutting and chopping food as it enters the mouth.

b. *Canine teeth*, or tusks − There is one in each interdental space, top and bottom, between the incisors and molars. They are usually only seen in the male. The lower pair are situated in front of the upper pair.

c. *Molars* − There are six on each side of both jaws − making 24 in all. They are large teeth with rough wearing surfaces and are responsible for grinding food.

d. *Wolf Teeth* − These are two in number and appear just in front of the first molar on each side of the upper jaw only. They are smaller than any other teeth and vary in size from little more than a pinhead to almost as big as a canine tooth. Because of their small size and shallow roots, they are easily moved by the pressure of a bit; this creates pain and may cause the horse to throw his head about when ridden. Wolf teeth are routinely removed as soon as they appear.

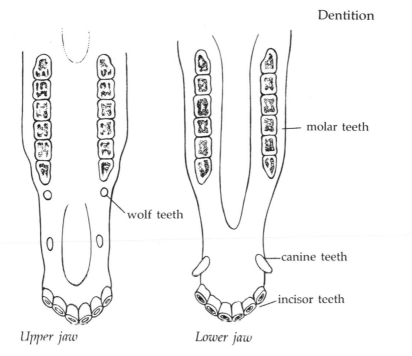

molar teeth

wolf teeth

canine teeth

incisor teeth

Upper jaw   *Lower jaw*

For the purpose of ageing a horse, most information is provided by the incisors.

The illustrations accompanying this section will make clear the difference between milk and permanent teeth. Up to five years of age the casting of the milk teeth and their replacement by permanents varies very little. After five, when all the incisors are permanent, it is necessary to rely on other signs, i.e. angles, shape, marks, etc.

These signs are not as accurate as the arrival of new teeth, but taken together, there should be no real difficulty in estimating the age of most horses to within a year or two.

The pattern of tooth change is as follows.

 a. A 2-year-old shows a full mouth of temporary incisors — six on both the top and bottom jaw. Owing to their whiteness and shape there should be no difficulty in differentiating them from permanent teeth.

 b. At 2½ to 3 years, the central pair of milk incisors are replaced by permanent teeth.

 c. At 3½ to 4 years, the lateral pair of milk teeth are replaced by permanent teeth.

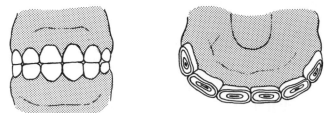

Two-year-old — all teeth are temporary

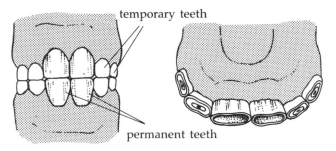

temporary teeth

permanent teeth

Three-year-old

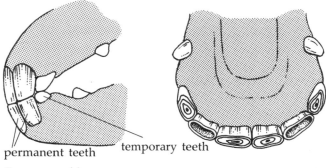

permanent teeth   temporary teeth

Four-year-old

    d. At 4½ to 5 years, the corner pair of milk teeth are replaced by permanent teeth.

    e. At 5 years, the corner incisors are not meeting fully, and are described as 'shelly'.

The horse now has a full mouth of permanent teeth and other signs must be taken into consideration.

    f. At 6 years, the corner teeth have worn level. The horse now has all incisor tables level and in wear.

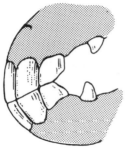

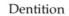

Five-year-old

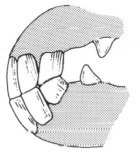

Six-year-old

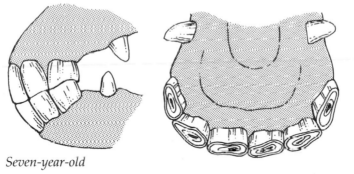

Seven-year-old

From this point on, the shape of the teeth, the wear of the infundibula — the cups or marks — and the presence of Galvayne's groove are taken into account.

    g. At 7 years, the cup in the table of the central incisors has often grown out but the outline remains. A hook is seen at the back of the upper corner incisor; this is due to the tooth not fully meeting its opposite number in the lower jaw.

h. At 8 years, the cup has worn out from the laterals but the outline remains. Between the outline of the cup and the front of
the tooth a further mark now appears in the form of a dark
line — known as the dental star. It is seen in the centrals at
this age. The 7-year-old hook has worn away.

i. At 9 years, the cups disappear from all the incisors, but the
outline will be evident at the corners. The dental star is distinct
on the laterals. At about this age a second hook develops on
the corner tooth. Unlike the 7-year-old hook, this is the direct
effect of wear.

j. At 10 years, the cups have gone and the dental star is distinct
on all incisors. The shape of the teeth now changes, the tables
becoming more triangular with age.

k. Another sign to assist ageing appears in the upper corner
incisors at 9 to 10 years. It is a dark groove, called Galvayne's
groove. It is on the outer surface of the tooth and commences
at the gum. By 15 years, it has reached half way down the
tooth and by 20 it extends the whole length.

As well as observing the dental stars appearing in place of the cups,
and the length of Galvayne's groove, it is important to watch the length
of the teeth and their angle to the jaw.

To summarise, a typical mouth will age as follows.

1-year-old: six white teeth in both jaws showing the typical neck of a
milk tooth. The corner teeth are not in full wear.

2-year-old: the same but with the corners in wear.

3-year-old: two central permanents in wear and four milk teeth outside
them on each row.

4-year-old: two central permanent teeth and one lateral on each side
of them, on each row.

5-year-old: a full mouth of permanent teeth, the laterals not in full wear.

6-year-old: a full mouth with all in wear, cups visible on all.

7-year-old: a full mouth, no cups in centrals, hook on outside of upper
corner incisor.

8-year-old: a full mouth, no cups on centrals or laterals, but a small
dark area appears on the tables of the centrals in place of
the cups, and the hook on the upper incisor disappears.

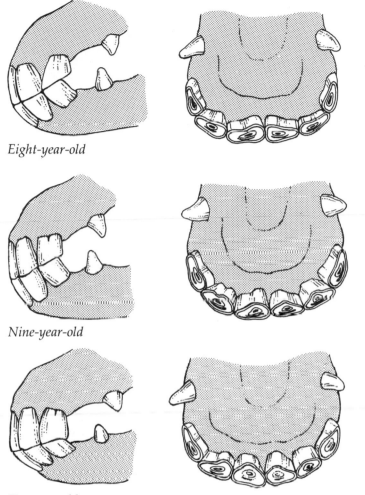

Eight-year-old

Nine-year-old

Ten-year-old

9-year-old: a full mouth, the centrals changing from oval to triangular. Galvayne's groove on upper corner incisor, dark spot on the tables of the centrals and laterals. A nine-year-old hook on the upper corner tooth.

10-year-old: a full mouth, dark spot on all lower incisors, centrals and laterals becoming more triangular, Galvayne's groove about 6 mm (¼ in.) long, lower and upper incisors starting to slope forward.

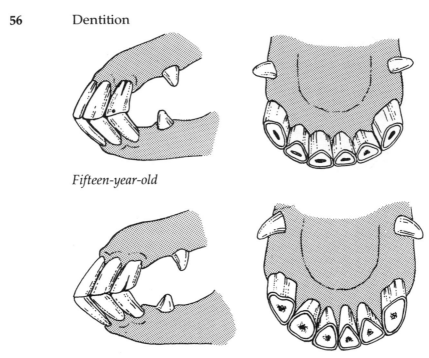

Fifteen-year-old

Twenty-year-old

11-year-old: a full mouth, all incisors assuming a triangular shape, Galvayne's groove 6 mm−1.8 cm (¼−¾ in.) long.

12-year-old ⎫
13-year-old ⎪ incisors triangular in shape, slope increasing, Galvayne's
14-year-old ⎬ groove growing by about 3 mm (⅛ in.) each year.
15-year-old ⎭

6 General Signs of Health and Disease

It is appropriate at this point to consider the general signs of health in order that symptoms of ill-health will be recognised when we consider disease. It has to be said that the recognition of illness in horses is something which is not a natural instinct; the signs are identified by a combination of observation and learning, which takes time and effort. It is not very simple, and the instincts which develop in time are really based on a great deal of thought and acquired experience.

In general the animal should be bright and alert with a normal posture and be in fair or good condition. Horses usually remain standing in the daytime, but a healthy horse lying down will normally get up when approached, unless he is very familiar with, and relaxed in the company of, the person approaching.

The coat of a horse at grass should lie flat and have a certain amount of gloss or sheen to it, except perhaps in winter, when the coat will be longer and the texture is affected by rain and mud. However, a horse wintered out should have a warmth to his skin and should hold condition. If he does not he may well need attention. Bald patches on the coat should be treated with suspicion; they may indicate infestation with lice or ringworm.

The skin should be loose on the underlying tissues and free from excessive scurf. A tight skin can signify dehydration in a horse in work.

The eye should be bright and full. When the lids are turned back the membranes should be a pale salmon-pink colour. There should be no sign of discharges.

The pulse can be taken on the inner surface of the lower jaw on either side. It is a measure of the heartbeat and can also indicate the strength at which the blood is being pumped through the circulation. In extreme illness the pulse may become weak and thready. In a fit animal at rest the pulse will be in the region of 35–40 per minute, or less, and will be described as full and strong.

The normal *rectal temperature* of a horse is 100−101.5 °F (37.7−38.6 °C).

Urine is very often colourless, but a great deal of variety is allowed under normal circumstances. The urine can be thick and cloudy in animals on high-quality feeds, and this does not have to be considered a sign of ill-health. Likewise mares in season have urine of a soupy consistency which may be passed with increased frequency and be almost white in colour. It is clear that urinary problems in the modern horse are far less common than they were thought to be by our ancestors.

The colour and consistency of *faeces* will vary with diet but they should be at all times moist, free of slime and offensive odours. Observation of droppings is an essential aspect of horsemanship, and it is important that any gross change in quantity, colour or texture be noted quickly.

The limbs should not be filled or swollen.

The respirations should be even and regular and at a rate of 8−12 per minute when the horse is at rest. Both the nostrils and ribs should make movements which are barely perceptible. The membranes of the nasal passages should be the same salmon-pink colour as those of the eye. There should be no discharges evident.

When eating long fodder the grind of the *teeth* should be even. The remains of food in the manger may give indications of problems with mastication. There may be saliva spilling from the mouth or 'balls' of undigested material scattered about.

The action and movement of a healthy horse should be sprightly and free when the horse is led in hand. While some animals are undoubtedly lazy and docile, the person looking after the animal should know their charge, appreciate any change in his normal state and thus recognise the line between health and illness.

In the field, an unhealthy horse may stand in one place if he is not eating. All of his vital functions need to be observed. Of course, he could simply be resting, but the distinction has to be made.

Where any variation occurs in the normal healthy signs, there are general indications of disease.

Sick animals generally appear listless. The head may be lowered with drooping ears. Gait and even posture may be unsteady. The horse may be in poor or bad condition, though this is not always the case.

The coat may be staring, or on end. It will appear dull and have lost its healthy bloom. There may be skin lesions. The coat and eye are considered by many to be the mirrors of health in the body.

Examine the *mane*. In good health the hair is firm and not easily pulled out. It may be broken and short where an animal has been scratching because of lice or sweet itch. With lice there may be extensive bare patches in the coat.

A *tight skin* is a sign of dehydration or, even worse, malnutrition. It will also be tight in the early stages of infectious diseases, where the animal may have dehydrated as a response to a persistent high temperature.

Excess *sweating* can result from too much exercise in unfit animals. It may also occur as a response to excitement. Light sweating is not uncommon with infection.

A *cold sweat* usually occurs when the animal is at rest, generally after exercise, but may also occur at other times. Whatever the cause, sweating in abnormal situations is very likely to be a sign of clinical problems and should always be treated accordingly.

Pale membranes denote anaemia. This may be caused by a number of factors, the most common of which is red worm, though it could be caused by haemorrhage — external or internal — or any factor which caused the process of building red cells to be disturbed.

Yellow membranes generally indicate disorders of the liver. There are many shades of this discolouration seen nowadays, especially in conditions such as herpes-virus infections.

Deep red or *injected membranes* may be caused by high temperatures, but they are evident as residual signs of virus infections.

Improper or inadequate oxygenation of the blood due to pneumonia causes the blood to become *darker* and the *membranes* may reflect this in their colour.

Blue membranes may indicate cardiac trouble, but they are also a feature of certain poisonings which interfere with oxygenation of the red cells, such as nitrite poisoning.

An increase of the *resting pulse* to 50 or over warrants further examination. It could mean the animal is in pain and starting a bout of colic. It could, equally, be a sign of developing fever. An irregularity of the beat generally indicates problems associated with the *heart*, though not all irregular patterns are necessarily clinical.

A rise in temperature of two or three degrees may accompany acute pain, but it could also be a sign of infection.

Before suspecting *urinary problems*, the animal should be seen to be in some discomfort when passing urine and urinating more than usual. A great deal of normal variation is allowed in healthy horses, but if there is suspicion that the animal is unwell further advice should be sought.

A certain amount of *faecal discolouration* is due to changes which may occur naturally in the composition of feed. If there are signs of *blood* or *mucus* they indicate damage to the lining of the bowel. If the *texture* suddenly changes this should be taken seriously. A great deal of large-bowel digestion is carried out by micro-organisms. If the balance of these organisms is disturbed, severe *scouring* may result which can be very difficult to control. It happens most often when there is a gross change in feed ingredients. It frequently happens in animals changed from poor to very lush pastures. *Offensive smells* are a sign of abnormality as the faeces of the horse are generally mildly odoured.

Filling of the legs may indicate circulatory problems. It may also be associated with digestive troubles. If confined to a single limb or joint, the cause is more likely to be lameness or local irritation.

Evident *increases in respiration* rate and effort are indicative of pain or infection. *Coughing* is a common sign of diseases such as *influenza*, and may also be a feature of broken wind. Horses with herpes infections of the upper respiratory tract tend to *blow their noses* forcefully with great frequency. With *strangles*, the first diagnostic sign of infection is a sore throat and difficulty in swallowing.

Horses which *quid their food* may have uneven molar tables with sharp edges which are irritating the gums.

7 Body Defences Against Disease and Injury

The defensive instincts of the animal body form a complex of weapons which are aimed to sustain life in the face of all the challenges it is likely to meet. In a hostile environment, such as the one we live in, there is constant danger, be it from micro-organisms which gain entry through the body systems, or broken skin, or larger predators which constantly question the pecking order of existence.

We have already referred briefly to the stay apparatus in the horse's legs. This is a system of tendons and ligaments which has a number of purposes one being to permit the horse to rest while standing, so that his escape from any surprise attack is quicker. Obviously this system, which interplays with other limb structures, was originally designed for life in the wild, but its very presence is an indication of the direction of evolution and the importance of defensive systems to the body at large.

The minute, even microscopic, defences are a great deal more complex than the stay apparatus and form a continuing battle-front that starts at every external opening and extends through to the blood, down as far as the substance of each body cell.

Externally, *the skin* is the first line of defence, but the *small hairs* which line the entrances to the nasal passages act as filters to foreign material entering in inhaled air. This filtering continues down along the respiratory tract, where hairs are replaced by hair-like extensions of the surface cells called *cilia*. These trap dirt or organisms which reach them, and their protection extends almost to the alveoli of the lungs. Because of *mucus* excreted by glands in the same linings, this dirt is trapped and removed to the outside through a wave-like motion of the surface which simply sweeps it out before it.

Then there are numerous *chemicals* which are immediate defences against organisms. The fluid that bathes the eye contains an enzyme called *lysozyme*. If organisms have passed the quick reflexes of the lids, and the filtering effects of lashes, they are then attacked by this enzyme, the purpose of which is to destroy and defend. There are similar enzymes in the mouth, and the acid in the stomach accounts for many organisms that travel that far.

The next line of defence stands against *bacteria* and *viruses* which have passed the outer defences and entered body cells and fluids. Here they are likely to be swallowed by scavenger white cells — *macrophages* — in the blood and tissue fluids, whose purpose is to envelop and destroy foreign material. However, as infection depends on the organism overcoming defences, it can happen that the defending cells are beaten. The organisms may well grow and multiply within them, despite an extensive armoury of chemical resistance, and then burst out releasing fresh infection into the tissues and blood.

The *white cells* of the blood then try to limit spread, and organisms are attacked in lymph glands, the liver, even within the circulation. The immune system is also in play at this stage, bringing with it antibodies and other chemicals to support the effort.

It is a tribute to the effectiveness of these systems that our animals so seldom die of infection — except at times when reduced resistance gives the organism greater advantage. This is the problem with many lethal infections of foals.

In infections such as equine flu the virus increases its virulence as an epidemic builds up. Rapid growth allows for the development of new varieties of virus, against which the body will have no defence, but, overall, the infection is eventually beaten and life returns to normal.

Immunity is divided into that which we are born with and that which develops as we encounter organisms through life. It is a subject of great complexity, but it is also a means we use — through vaccination — to defend animals against known infections. Some vaccines are more effective than others but science is constantly learning and working for the future. Because of the nature and small size of viruses, vaccines are less effective against them than against bacteria. Vaccination against tetanus — a bacterial infection — is very effective, while vaccination against flu is sometimes disappointing.

The body's *response to injury* is equally well organised. Fluid is poured into damaged areas carrying with it the cells which organise repair. The effect of this is to create swelling, thereby limiting movement. The cells also digest and remove damaged tissue. The external signs of injury are *heat*, *pain* and *swelling*.

The swelling allows the part to be repaired without being subjected to further damage. Pain is also a positive response of the body to protect the injured part. It is wrong to suppress pain if doing so allows the tissues to be used and so become more seriously hurt.

The *blood supply* to an injured area is increased, bringing with it all the materials necessary for repair. A lymph-type fluid is poured out of blood vessel walls accompanied by large numbers of white cells. These cells attack bacteria, viruses or physical dirt which may have found a way into the injured tissues. They also digest and remove damaged tissue. If injury includes rupture of vessels, the result is a greater out-pouring and there will be whole blood present. Pain is caused by pressure on local nerve endings as well as direct damage suffered by nerves in the locality. Subsequently, it is usually movement of the injury that causes most acute pain.

The inflammatory response is always an answer to a challenge, be it *mechanical*, *chemical*, or *infectious*. From the patient's point of view, it is designed to limit damage and foster repair. It is not a negative or harmful reaction but a designed effort which is of considerable benefit.

In certain situations, however, the progress of the repair process is less than perfect. Different factors can convert an *acute reaction* into a *chronic* one, and, while the damage may be limited, an area may be left which is not restored to full functional health. For example:

a. Repair of small injuries to the sesamoid bones is limited by the forces pulling the injured parts away from one another. While the body will pour fluid in to fill the gap and attempt to organise the repair, it is physically unable to overcome the handicap. Assistance will have to be given to the tissues to effect a full recovery.

b. In muscular injuries, the injured muscle very often is taken out of use and its place compensated for by the other muscles surrounding it. However, it is vital to the repair of the injured tissues that they be encouraged to come back into use; this the body is very often unable to do.

c. In damage to areas where different tissues are in apposition the repair may leave adhesions between these tissues, thereby limiting movement. This can happen when tendons are damaged. The presence of adhesions reduce the chance of a horse returning to working soundness.

It is therefore the purpose of any treatment of physically damaged tissues to *guide* and *control* the inflammatory processes rather than inhibit them. While there are situations where the use of anti-inflammatory drugs such as corticosteroids is indicated, that decision will be made by a veterinary surgeon, depending on the circumstances. The limitation of pain and support of injured areas is a prime consideration in all situations, but the ultimate aim is repair and return of full use to the part.

Invariably there is a halfway point between the ideal and what is necessary. An irreparably damaged horse has to be put out of pain. However drugs that kill pain may be used in the initial stages to *relieve suffering* if there is a chance of recovery, and anti-inflammatory drugs may have a part to play here too.

The *aim of repair* is to encourage the absorption of dead cells and blood clots and return full mobility to a part. *Bleeding* must be limited as far as possible, even by the use of external pressure bandages − the degree of swelling is kept within limits by the same procedure. *Cold* applications constrict blood vessels and limit the flow of blood into an area. Some advocate the use of hot dressings at this point − or alternate hot and cold dressings − but the benefit of this is disputed. Most modern approaches tend to aim at the use of cold rather than heat, except where there is danger of local infection when hot poultices are used routinely. To apply heat to already damaged tissue may defeat the aim of controlling the influx of fluid. Cold applications need to be continued for long periods to be effective.

Support for the area is important, when it can be done. This applies mostly to the lower limbs. The aim is to limit swelling and assist the venous circulation to evacuate the area. Pain is controlled in the process, partly by reducing movement of the injury.

Once the initial condition has stabilised, i.e. when swelling is controlled and pain is limited, a different approach to repair can be taken. *Physiotherapy* in varions forms can be started. The purpose of physiotherapy is to restore function to the part and promote healing by purely physical means. This can vary from simple massage to the use of modern electrical equipment which has a deeper, but similar, effect. More will be said of these later.

Until now, *firing* and *blistering* were used as a form of counter-irritation to stimulate repair of chronic injuries which had not responded to other therapy. The technique involved the application of an irritant — either chemical or actual heat — to the skin, causing an influx of fluid and cells to the area. There is a body of opinion still in favour of the practice, but it would be hard to say that these methods have any advantage over more humane modern therapies. Thankfully, firing is now being banned by the Royal College of Veterinary surgeons.

When blisters are used the following points should be kept in mind:

a. The diet should be reduced prior to treatment as part of the letting-down process, except where a very mild working blister is being used while an animal is still in work.

b. Areas such as the hollow of the heels and backs of the knees should be coated in vaseline to protect them from the effects of the blister.

c. If a foreleg is being blistered, both legs should be done to prevent too much weight being borne by the good leg. If only one leg is blistered a strong supporting bandage should be applied to the other for the same reason.

d. No blister should be applied to an acutely injured area.

8 Repair and Treatment of Wounds

Wounds may be divided into the following categories, always remembering that infinite variations occur and no two wounds are ever the same.

a. *Abrasions* — only the surface of the skin is damaged and sensitive areas are exposed. They may result from falls on hard surfaces, scraping legs while being loaded onto a trailer or from minor overreaches and brushing.

b. *Simple skin wounds* caused by sharp instruments. The wound is clean and free from contamination.

c. *Contusions* occur from falls, kicks, etc. The skin is broken but the edges of the wound do not part.

d. *Lacerations* with damage to deeper tissues. The edges of the wound are irregular and there is usually a certain amount of dead tissue.

e. *Puncture wounds*.

f. Where there is *complete loss* of *skin* from an area.

Repair

In a simple wound caused by a surgeon's knife there is a deliberate attempt made to avoid infection and keep the wound clean. The knife will have been sterilised and the skin treated with bactericidal solutions. Therefore, under ideal circumstances, the wound will heal without infection. The process through which this happens is as follows.

Bleeding occurs into the incision and the blood *clots*. As the clot shrinks, the sides of the wound are drawn together and held there by the glue-like properties of the coagulum. *White cells* invade this and gradually digest it. *Connective tissue* cells multiply and *small blood vessels* invade the area. The purpose of this is to strengthen the repair and provide a new circulation to replace damaged vessels. *Surface cells* proliferate and close the incision. The complete process will take about one week to ten days.

There is *no discharge* from such a wound unless irritants are applied mistakenly to clean it. However, if organisms are introduced, the area becomes inflamed and there will be discharges and local tissue swelling. If the wound has been stitched the reaction will be greater because of inadequate drainage.

Infected wounds heal by granulation — this is the most common form of healing we see. It is based on a combination of fibrous tissue and blood vessels. White cells come in and attack any foreign matter in the wound. Once this process is completed and the wound is fully filled by new tissue, the wound becomes impervious to further infection. Surface cells will then grow and cover the new tissue which gradually retreats as the healing process is completed.

Where there is excessive movement on a wound, e.g. a transverse wound on the front of the knee, or where the two ends of the wound are being dragged apart by gravity, etc., there is delayed healing and very often *proud flesh*.

Treatment

Because of the variety of wounds, it is not easy to generalise on treatment, but some basic principles apply.

a. The danger of infection exists with all wounds. As the organism causing *tetanus* is a common contaminant it is advisable to make sure that the animal is covered either through vaccination or with anti-serum.

b. *First-aid* principles demand the control of bleeding and support of damaged tissues. This may be effected by applying pressure to exposed bleeding points and bandaging the area until treatment can proceed.

c. The next requirement is to make sure the *wound* is *clean*. All visible dirt must be picked out, but this may only be possible under local anaesthetic and it then becomes a job for the veterinary surgeon. Only very mild, warm solutions should be used for cleaning as more irritant antiseptics will further damage exposed tissues and complicate healing. Boiling water will do the same. No strong antiseptics or disinfectants should be used unless greatly diluted.

d. If the wound is clean and is not in need of stitching it may be advisable to *cover* it if possible. This is done for two reasons: firstly, to limit effusion of body fluid into the area; secondly, to support the damaged structures and help them to stay in apposition (i.e. direct and level contact) as they knit. A dressing of wound powder should be applied first followed by some sterile cotton wool or gauze. An outer layer of adhesive bandage helps to hold the dressing in place.

There comes a point, after the initial body reaction has been stemmed, when the wound will benefit from *exposure to air*. At this stage a powder may be applied locally to help drying and keep the surface from invasion.

e. In badly *infected wounds* it may be necessary to apply poultices, change dressings regularly, and use injections of antibiotics to control the problem. To an extent, strong supporting dressings will, through the application of pressure, limit proud flesh.

f. Where there is a sign of *delayed healing*, or proud flesh formation, use of physiotherapy is very effective in promoting good union and stemming excessive growth. Using either ultrasound or lasers − once infection has been overcome − the reaction stimulates strong growth at the edge of the wound and early control of granulation. There are also drugs available which assist this process, although perhaps not as effectively as physiotherapy.

g. Wounds and abrasions which are left open from the start may be treated locally with a suitable *wound powder* or spray. The main purpose of these will be to kill surface organisms and allow healing.

h. With infected wounds it may be necessary to *replace dressings* every 12 or 24 hours. On removing the dressing a yellow sticky mass will be seen. This should be gently cleaned away using swabs of cotton wool dipped in warm saline solution or one containing well-diluted antiseptics. The point of the exercise is to help the body by getting rid of the discharges. However it is not advisable to be too vigorous as it is possible to damage the delicate processes in hand.

i. If there is *dead tissue* this may need to be removed. Flaps of skin which have been cut off from their blood supply are unable to survive and will shrivel up. A veterinary surgeon will decide if these are to be surgically removed. However in very obvious cases they can be cut off with a blade or scissors. The important thing is to seek advice if in doubt.

j. Where the edges of a wound are being *pulled apart* by natural dynamic factors – as in all transverse limb wounds – it is vital to limit movement. This may be effected by applying bandages which support the tissues and keep the ends together. Alternatively, something stronger like a cast or splint may have the same effect, although the total exclusion of drainage and air is not beneficial, particularly in infected wounds. This may be overcome to an extent by the use of a window in the cast, allowing the movement to be prevented and the wound cleaned.

k. *Puncture wounds* require the use of antibiotics, both locally and by injection. It is important also to draw infected material to the surface with poultices. If this is not achieved there is a danger of abscess formation.

l. Where *thorns* have penetrated deeply into tissues, unless they can be seen and withdrawn, there will be a constant chronic reaction which will not heal. Continuous poulticing may draw the wound, or it may be possible to lance the tissues and force the thorn out. Pieces of glass may remain in tissues for years.

m. Always encourage *drainage* and if bathing is necessary – particularly where infection has moved away from the opening – bathe towards the opening.

n. Where *exudate* is passively travelling under the skin down the leg it is important to limit infection. Occasionally added drainage points have to be created surgically to allow infected matter to escape.

o. Exercise is important from the time a wound is strong enough to withstand it. This may be confined to a short walk about the box or yard. It helps to strengthen the repair and leave a wound which will not break down when the animal is returned to work.

p. With puncture wounds of the *foot* an exception is made to the advice regarding strong antiseptics and disinfectants. It is advisable to dip the foot into a strong solution which will help to kill infection. This is assisted by increasing *drainage* where needed, but only as far as is essential — too vigorous cutting can harm the sensitive tissues underneath. It is then best to apply a poultice. Where proud flesh appears on the foot, it may have to be burned off with a caustic, such as copper sulphate powder. Five per cent solutions of copper sulphate may be used for less radical treatment of infections such as thrush.

q. Where a wound involves a *bursa* or *joint* the use of antibiotics is critical to control infection. *Ultrasound* is also useful in getting the bursa or joint to close — once infection has been repelled — so allowing the outer wound to follow suit. Physiotherapy not only limits the development of adhesions but can help those already existing to be broken down.

r. Virtually all leg wounds cause damage to circulation. This will result in *filling* of the leg until the situation returns to normality. Where a *major vein* has been seriously damaged, collateral circulation has to be established. This is sometimes evident on the neck when a jugular vein has been obliterated. A mesh of small veins may appear in the area, which take over the drainage of local tissues. Such an event in a leg wound can take a considerable time to mend. Controlled exercise is important to hasten the process.

s. Where a wound overlies bone it is important to ensure that the bone itself is not damaged — using x-rays if necessary.

t. *Overreaches* occur on the bulbs of the heel and at the back of the fetlock joint. Healing is often slow, but the same general principles apply as were mentioned for indolent (slow to heal) wounds.

u. Where the *flexor tendons* are damaged during self-inflicted injuries, it is advisable to treat the problem with extreme caution. While the surface wound may be insignificant the damage to deeper tissues can be serious. The wound should seldom be stitched, and infection dealt with as above. The damage to the tendon can only be estimated in the light of day. Professional advice is strongly advised.

v. Injuries to the *coronary band* respond well to *ultrasound* therapy.

w. Animals which injure themselves by *stumbling* often have an underlying problem. It may have to do with the balance of the legs and is often correctable.

x. Where there is total *loss of skin* from an area the animal's ability to survive will depend on the extent. In some cases an early decision will have to be made to destroy the animal.

However, where the area is of a manageable size — and this decision may have to be made by a professional person — the important thing is to stem the outflow of serous fluid, to protect the area from contamination, and encourage the edges of skin to close over by degrees. It is remarkable how many big wounds heal successfully and leave quite tidy scarring.

9　Infectious Disease

A great part of the efforts of the modern equine veterinary surgeon is spent on the treatment of infectious conditions. While a certain amount of these fall into specific categories — e.g. strangles, a bacterial disease, or equine influenza, caused by a virus — many are not easily labelled. Most bacterial conditions, in fact, fall into a range of non-specific chills and infections which respond to antibiotic treatment and are not identified. Infected wounds generally contain mixed organisms and the only point in identifying these is to locate a suitable antibiotic if they fail to respond to treatment. There is seldom time to do this in the average infection, because immediate treatment has to be started.

Bacteria are single-cell organisms which reproduce by simple division, and are widely distributed in nature. They are readily seen under a microscope at magnifications of about 1000. They grow with ease in decomposed animal or human matter. There are varieties which live in soil, others which are vital to natural processes such as digestion; and some which inhabit the surfaces of the body.

From a disease viewpoint, there are bacteria that need oxygen for growth and those that thrive best in areas devoid of it, like dead and decaying tissues. Many bacteria, though not primary causes of disease, are able to set up infection if in contact with tissues which have already been debilitated.

Infection is simply an invasion of tissues which are then used as a basis for further growth and multiplication. In septicaemia, the bacteria invade the bloodstream and spread throughout the body. This, as might be expected, is very serious. It may occur as an extension from other infections, of, say, the bowel or respiratory system.

Bacteria vary greatly in their ability to set up disease. However the simple presence of an organism does not have to mean disease, because, as was explained earlier, there is first a battle with the body defences, and the organism may well be defeated.

Bacteria are commonly *cultured* from uterine infections of mares, from infected discharges, and from the rectum of foals with scours.

In such cases a swab is taken. For uterine infections the swab is taken from the mare's cervix. The swab consists of sterile cotton wool attached to a probe. It is brought into direct contact with the open cervix where it absorbs some of the fluid emerging from the uterus. The swab must not touch any other tissue; even touching a freshly washed hand will contaminate the swab. When taken, it is placed in a sterile container, which will usually contain a transport medium. This medium will prevent the cotton wool from drying, and encourage growth of any organisms contained in it.

At the laboratory, the swab is smeared onto a plate of sterile culture material, such as *blood agar*, and placed into an *incubator*. Within 24 hours, an infected swab will produce a growth in most cases. The organism can then be identified and a *sensitivity test* carried out to discover which antibiotics will be most effective against it. This is done by laying a fresh growth onto another plate containing numerous small discs of different *antibiotics*. The bacteria will gradually invade the areas around those discs to which they are resistant. Clear areas indicate that the organism is vulnerable to antibiotics in the related discs. The animal is then treated on the basis of this information.

In acute foal scours, it is not possible to wait for test results, so treatment has to be started immediately. However a result may be available by the time further treatment is needed and this can be of benefit.

It is important that any bacterial infection is terminated as soon as possible in order to limit the damage done to animal tissues. There are, however, many situations in which it is not easy to take a swab. In these instances, the treating veterinary surgeon has to rely on his knowledge and instincts to reach a cure.

Paths of Infection

As indicated earlier, bacteria have to enter the body through the existing natural openings, or through the broken skin. It is important to understand that bacteria are so widely available in nature that injured or damaged tissues are easy prey to them. It is for this reason hygiene is so critical. We must understand the nature of infection if we are to contain it. This is particularly so when we are dealing with highly contagious conditions such as *strangles*, and highly infectious ones such as *anthrax*. 'Infectious' means that the organism will inevitably set up infection when it enters the body. 'Contagious' means it is readily spread.

Contagious infection finds an easy path from one animal to another. For example, strangles, which is passed on by the discharges coming from infected horses. If these get onto a field, all other horses which subsequently graze it may pick up the infection. The contact can also be made through human agencies. It can be carried on hands and clothing, transported on or in, buckets and other implements, food sacks, muck sacks, etc. Remembering this is critical to control of the disease.

Anthrax is a highly *infectious* condition that is spread from contaminated sources, such as improperly sterilised meat and bone meal. It is also present in soil. Animals found to have died from it are buried on the spot under conditions which give the infection no chance to spread further.

Although anthrax is lethal it is relatively uncommon in horses. Alas, strangles is not uncommon, though it kills few animals. Anthrax is said to have a high *mortality* but low *morbidity*, i.e. relatively few animals affected. Strangles is the opposite.

Once inside the body, organisms are in a position to set up infection if the opportunity arises. If resistance is lowered, either through poor nutrition, management mistakes, etc., infection is the natural sequel. Removing one organism may only give opportunity to others if the underlying problem is not solved.

Steps for Controlling Infection

a. Make sure the animal is well nourished. Malnutrition lowers disease resistance.

b. Ensure stabling is warm, dry and clean.

c. Containers and utensils must be clean at all times, e.g. feed bowls, and water buckets and bowls. Any waste food and animal discharges will be a fertile medium for organisms to grow on. Inhaled into the respiratory system these may lead to pneumonia. In the gut they can compete with beneficial organisms and lead to acute infections of the bowel.

d. The feed room must be scrupulously clean and the method of distributing food to large numbers of horses must be hygienic as well as efficient. If sacks are used they should be washed regularly.
e. Hands, grooming kit and tack must be kept clean. Remember that highly contagious conditions like ringworm are spread by these means.
f. The boots of stable workers may be a source of disease spreading. It is wise to have disinfectant outside stables in order that boots can be dipped between infected horses. This is good practice in any serious outbreak of infection.
g. Vehicles going out of, or coming into, a yard may carry infection. In major outbreaks, disinfectant pads outside the yard gates will need to be long enough to take a full revolution of the wheels.

Virus Infections

The most noteworthy differences between bacteria and viruses are the much *smaller size* of virus particles, and the way they live. Viruses are not complete in themselves. They cannot live and reproduce except in the substance of a *living cell*. They do not survive for long in nature.

A virus needs the material of a living cell to allow it to grow and multiply. Outside the body it is subject to death from drying, heat, exposure to the sun, etc. It may live for a limited time in discharges which protect it from these hazards. It is preserved, to a degree, by freezing. However it has to get back into living tissue to continue existing.

Viruses have to face the same defensive systems as bacteria. Their great advantage is their small size, which allows easy penetration to the deeper tissues of the lungs in inhaled air — this is their most common portal of entry. They also have the ability to grow rapidly and constantly produce new varieties by a process called *mutation*. This poses great problems for the defence systems.

On the other hand, viruses, while often tending to be very contagious are not always highly infectious. In many cases their ability to set up disease is dependent on a lowering of the resistance of the host. Their most common cycle of infection is short — a matter of days — but this is extended by the host's weakness or any external factor that contributes to it.

The spread of a virus is much the same as for bacteria, with one major difference; it is contained in discharges which may be picked up by hands, clothing, etc., but the most important spread is *in air* contaminated with infected respiratory discharges. When coughed or blown out of the nasal passages, viruses will travel for varying distances depending on particle size. The influenza virus will be coughed directly into the air and so reach other horses in an immediate building, or at a sale, meeting or event. This virus will not, unlike the herpes virus that causes rhinopneumonitis and abortion in mares, travel over longer distances on the wind. The herpes virus can travel 20 miles or more in air, this is a major factor in the spread of the disease. Horses cough little with the herpes virus, though they clear their noses in an explosive way that has a similar effect.

Specific Infections

Strangles

This disease is restricted to equines. It is highly contagious, and the principle symptoms are a thick pustular discharge from the nostrils and gross enlargement of the glands under the back of the jaw. It can infect horses of all ages. After infection immunity is developed.

Strangles is spread through discharges. This may occur from animal to animal, and may also occur through human transportation on hands and equipment.

The condition is bacterial and once symptoms have begun to show the course is not easy to control. Swollen glands may break out and discharge pus for weeks on end.

Symptoms: The incubation period is in the region of 7−10 days, though it is reported as being shorter in established outbreaks. The first signs of the condition are an evident soreness of the throat with difficulty in swallowing. The horses make characteristic throaty sounds and may be unable to swallow solid food; they may even be disinclined to drink. The temperature rises to as high as 106 degrees and within days a watery discharge turns purulent at the nostrils. The submaxillary glands begin to swell. These swellings become hot, tense and painful, and may be

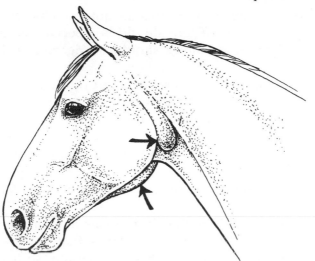

Enlarged glands in strangles

on one or both sides of the jaw. Other glands in the region may also become affected. The glands tend to burst and discharge pus and this may be a prolonged process, though complete recovery, after gland discharge, is frequent.

Diagnosis: The signs of painful throat with difficulty in swallowing is typical of early strangles infection and should be taken as a warning if seen in more than one animal at the time. The full course of the disease, with discharging glands etc., is easily recognised. Occasional cases of a similar type of infection occur in individual animals, not in whole herds. The organism causing the infection can be identified at a laboratory.

Treatment: Owing to the highly contagious nature of the disease, great care must be taken to isolate infected animals and prevent spread within a yard through utensils and vessels. If the first affected animal has managed to infect a pasture, it is advisable to suspend use of that pasture. Infection in stabled horses can occur only through direct contact and human assistance, therefore tight control on this is essential. Discharges from infected animals are potentially dangerous, so hands, clothing and footwear are in need of scrupulous attention. There should be containers of strong disinfectant outside stable doors for the feet of workers. Where possible a person attending an infected horse should not attend any other. However, if this is not possible the infected animal should be seen to last. There should be special feed and water buckets for each animal, and stables should be rigorously disinfected between horses.

Infected horses should be kept warm and out of draughts. Soft food and mashes are given to those with difficulty swallowing. Occasionally infection may invade the glands lining the bowel, and in these cases the outlook is guarded.

While penicillin is effective against the causal organism its use in an outbreak is of doubtful value. Although a vaccine has been produced, it is inclined to cause tissue reactions and has not been widely used in practice here.

The disease can be very debilitating and horses may take a long time to recover condition fully after an attack. Foals that get infection are more likely to die from septicaemia. This is especially so if the foal is in the first weeks of life.

Tetanus

This infection is very often lethal. The organism causing it enters the body through the broken skin. It inhabits the soil as a spore − a particularly durable phase in which it cannot reproduce − where it can remain for years. These spores can withstand boiling for up to an hour and are highly resistant to mild disinfectants.

On entering a wound the spore sheds its outer protective coat and begins to propagate in dead tissue when oxygen is excluded. During growth it produces a toxin which affects nerves and travels along them towards the central nervous system. It may also be carried in the lymph or blood. The symptoms depend on the amount of toxin and the parts of the nervous system affected. The incubation period varies from three days to three weeks, or longer. In some cases no wound is found.

Tetanus is an example of a disease which is highly infectious but not contagious.

Symptoms: These vary with the amount of toxin produced. There is rigidity of the limbs and the nictitating membrane − or haw − may be seen crossing the eye when the head is raised. The horse has trouble moving or holding his balance. He may not be able to eat from the ground, or swallow. There is a tendency for muscular spasm to occur

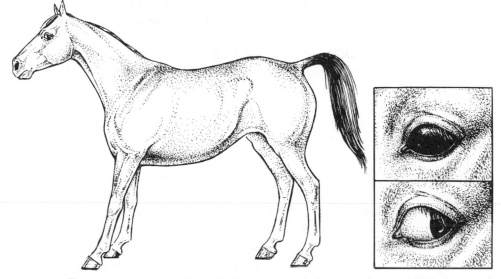

Tetanus symptoms: the typical stance, and the normal eye (above) compared to the eye of a tetanus-infected horse with the nictitating membrane, or haw, covering the eye (below).

and this is progressive. Reflexes are exaggerated, and because affected horses tend to topple over, they are kept in the dark – away from human and animal movement.

The horse may be unable to swallow because of spasm of the muscles of the head and neck. There may be frothing and nasal discharges – which may include the return of food materials down the nose. The animal is very apprehensive. Nostrils are often dilated, the lips drawn back with teeth exposed. The tail may be held up and seen to quiver. There may be profuse sweating, constipation, and urine may not be passed.

The rapidity with which symptoms develop will decide the outcome. If the horse goes down the prognosis is increasingly guarded.

Diagnosis: The progressive muscular rigidity is unmistakeable. The stance of affected animals is typical of tetanus. The term *lockjaw* describes how the muscles of the head are involved.

Treatment: The organism is sensitive to penicillin and the toxin is countered by anti-serum – though this is restricted once the toxin is affecting the nervous system. The chance of recovery in all cases of tetanus is not high, although some do return to normality. If the wound can be located, it should be drawn and cleaned out, using strong disinfectants if necessary.

Large doses of both drugs are used and repeated regularly. Soluble penicillin should be given intravenously every 12 hours. There are disagreements about the effectiveness of continued doses of serum, but these are often used in practice. Sedation may be necessary as may muscle-relaxant drugs in severe cases. While there is a danger in giving continuous doses of serum, very often the chance has to be taken.

The horse has to be nourished while recovering and body fluid levels maintained. Liquid food containing milk, eggs and electrolytes may be given by drench or stomach tube, though the risk of causing the animal to fall has to be considered. Sedation may be necessary at the time. Intravenous fluid therapy may be required.

Even when an animal is cured, the course of the disease is long, and full convalescence may take months.

Prevention: Today's vaccines are so effective that it is unusual to see tetanus in a vaccinated animal. Where there is doubt about vaccine status, a single injection of anti-serum should be given when any wound occurs. This will invariably prevent the development of symptoms.

Vaccination is effected by means of two injections, one month to six weeks apart. Immunity does not develop until about two weeks after the second injection. A booster is given after ten to twelve months, followed by further doses every two to three years. It is important to keep records of vaccination that will remain with the horse during the course of his life. If there is any doubt about the vaccinal status of a purchased animal there is no harm in providing him with a fresh course of injections. Foal vaccination is not usually started until about six months of life because maternal antibodies provided at birth may interfere. However at all times of risk anti-serum should be given.

Rhodococcus Infection of Foals

This is a bacterial infection of foals causing pneumonia. The organism is able to live in soil and dust and is not affected by direct sunlight. It is inhaled or eaten and is mainly noted for infecting foals in the first three months of life. Infection may well relate to lowered immunity or disease resistance, as older animals are seldom affected. It is marked by the development of abscesses in affected organs. Diagnosis is dependent on presentation of blood samples and materials for culturing to the laboratory. Antibiotics have an effect but their use may have to be greatly prolonged and the results are not always satisfactory.

Contagious Equine Metritis (CEM)

This is a bacterial disease of mares, affecting the reproductive organs, which first made an appearance in the 1970s. It is highly contagious and extremely virulent, causing profuse watery discharges to run down the quarters and legs of affected mares. Identification of the causal organism was made at the time, and a compulsory system of control was applied through the studs. Swabs were initially taken from the cervix and clitoris and these had to be clear of the organism before breeding was allowed. Stallions were similarly swabbed from the urethra and prepuce.

The incidence of infected swabs is now minimal, although precautions are still being taken.

The disease is notifiable.

Although the organism causing this disease has not been found in Thoroughbred mares in the past breeding season (1990), there is still concern about a low level of infection in non-thoroughbreds in both the United Kingdom and France. It is also known to exist in a number of other European countries.

A comprehensive Code of Practice exists, full details of which are available on request from the breeders' associations of any of the five participating countries – France, Germany, Ireland, Italy and the United Kingdom. The purpose of the code is to control equine venereal disease generally and to keep a constant check on new disease developments. It is important that this effort is respected and its minimum recommendations adhered to.

Fistulous Withers

This is a condition which has reduced greatly in incidence since the gradual elimination of brucellosis – the cause of abortion – from cattle. It consists of a pustular infection of the tissues in and around the withers. It is particularly difficult to treat because of the nature of the area and the lack of natural drainage. However, vaccination against brucellosis, although capable of causing considerable tissue reaction at the point of injection, can be very effective in curing the condition completely.

Poll Evil

Poll Evil is seldom seen nowadays and this may be for the same reason as the disappearance of fistulous withers. The condition is similar in nature except it occurs in the region of the poll, just behind the ears.

Fungal Diseases

Ringworm

Ringworm is a contagious disease caused by fungi. Circular areas of hair become raised, and a small amount of fluid exudes from the skin. The hair becomes matted and falls out, leaving a bald patch covered with dry greyish scales. These areas extend outward, usually retaining the circular shape. Because the fungus lives under the scales, the condition may have spread before being noticed.

Diagnosis: This is made on the basis of the symptoms and confirmed by skin scrapings submitted for laboratory examination.

Treatment: The treatment of choice is griseofulvin, given daily in the feed. However it is important to clean rugs and tack to prevent the spread of the condition. Some local sprays and washes are available, but for badly affected animals it is best to use griseofulvin.

The control of spread is critical. Hands, tack and implements are the most likely source. Some varieties of ringworm are transmissible to humans.

The following conditions are listed as notifiable under the Infectious Diseases of Horses Order, 1987:

    a. African Horse Sickness.
    b. Contagious Equine Metritis.
    c. Dourine.
    d. Epizootic Lymphangitis.
    e. Equine Infectious Anaemia.
    f. Equine Viral Encephalomyelitis.
    g. Glanders.

10   Virus Diseases

Equine Influenza

This is a virus disease of horses causing regular epidemics here. It is the only equine disease for which there is compulsory vaccination at present. It tends to become virulent in cycles with about 8–9 year intervals.

The virus has an almost worldwide distribution and was the cause of a major outbreak in Britain in 1989/90. There are three varieties named; A Equi/1 (Prague 56), A Equi/2 (Miami 63) and A Equi/2 (Kentucky 81) – the names indicating the source of the original virus isolation.

Infection in an animal is subject to the following:

a. Immune status. Not all vaccinated animals are adequately protected in the face of infection and there are numerous breakdowns reported. Better vaccines may soon be available.

b. Virulence of the virus. This grows as an outbreak gets under way.

c. The level of exposure. A small dose of the virus may be overcome by the body defences, but a massive dose will lead to inevitable infection unless there is solid immunity.

d. Environmental conditions play a part in infection. Conditions which are too cold or damp will hinder resistance and assist invasion.

e. Spread is mainly by droplet infection. As an infected horse coughs out virus it is inhaled directly into the lungs of another. Droplets are considered to travel about 20–30 m from the coughing animal.

f. The virus does not live for very long when outside the host but may be carried on contaminated clothing, hands, etc.

Symptoms: The virus affects old and young animals after an incubation period of as little as 1—3 days. There is a dry cough and a temperature as high as 106 °F. The horse will be off his food, depressed in appearance, and will develop a dirty nasal discharge. During the acute phase the animal is infectious to others — generally for 3—6 days. The cough may persist for several weeks. Pneumonia is a common secondary complication, especially in foals.

Diagnosis: The highly infectious nature of the condition, coughing and nasal discharges are confirmation of influenza. The virus can be isolated in a suitable laboratory.

Treatment: Antibiotics are used to control secondary infections. While these will not influence the viral phase of disease, they will help to shorten the overall length of illness and are vital in saving young animals from the effects of bacterial pneumonia.

It is advised to rest affected animals and restore lost weight fully before returning to work.

Prevention: Vaccination is compulsory for all animals taking part in racing. It is also made compulsory by the rules of individual organisations and competitions. All horses appearing on racecourses or at point-to-points are obliged to have a passport containing vaccination details.

While there are a number of vaccine types available, no preference is given to any one under Jockey Club rules. Neither is any advantage recorded in practice, though oil-based vaccines are more likely to cause local tissue reactions than water-based ones.

As the vaccines in use are live virus vaccines they create immunity by setting up a mild clinical infection. Because of this, vaccinated animals should be eased out of work for several days after having the injection.

The current regulations for vaccination under Jockey Club rules are:

a. Two initial injections to be given no less than 21 days apart and no longer than 92 days.
b. For horses foaled in 1980 or thereafter, a booster injection at not less than 150 days and not more than 215 days after the second initial dose.

c. Annual boosters at not more than a year apart. Prior to 16th March 1981, the period may have been one of 14 months.
d. No injection may have been given within seven days of a horse entering racecourse property.

Foals are not normally vaccinated until at least 3–6 months of age.

Herpes Virus Infection (Rhinopneumonitis)

This disease has assumed considerable modern importance as a cause of abortion in mares and respiratory infection in horses of all ages. It is also the cause of staggering, recumbency and paralysis in some horses. Severe outbreaks of this latter condition have occurred repeatedly over the past twenty years, mainly on stud farms. The respiratory disease is one of the main causes of concern to racehorse trainers.

Herpes viruses are considered to have a lifetime persistence in the body after infection, though there is some dispute as to the significance of this in horses. While, in particular instances, infection appears to carry on over a lengthy period, horses generally recover fully and are not chronically reinfected for the rest of their lives. However, reinfection may well ensue where resistance is lowered as this group of viruses is adept at exploiting any weakness in defence systems.

Herpes viruses are very fragile in nature and do not persist for very long on exposure. They are spread mainly by droplet infection and direct contact with contaminated material. Being extremely small the virus is spread over very wide areas on the wind. Almost all horses in a yard are infected quickly with the respiratory form of the disease.

Equine Herpes Virus 1 (EHV 1)

This is the cause of abortion in mares and upper respiratory disease in horses of all ages. It is a feature of the respiratory form that the infection can be persistent and extend to deeper organs of the body. The liver is commonly affected and the paralytic form of the disease is caused by this virus. Foals may be weak at birth and die in the first days of life. Pneumonia is a complication in older foals.

The virus is worldwide in distribution and is recognised as having been in existence throughout modern history.

Respiratory Form

Symptoms: After an incubation period of 2–10 days, there is a copious watery discharge from the nostrils. Horses will be heard clearing their noses in an explosive way that sprays infected material into the atmosphere as if sprayed from an aerosol. The virus can become very virulent where large numbers of horses are kept together.

High temperatures are possible in the early stages, though their duration may be short-lived — as little as 12 hours — and it is possible to miss them. There is depression, loss of appetite and the glands of the throat may be found to be swollen — though not to the degree of swelling with strangles. The membranes of the nasal passages acquire a typical purple discolouration. It is possible to miss the early signs.

In foals, pneumonia is a common outcome of this disease. While the general mortality rate is low, deaths may be common where the organism is virulent and management of a low order.

Systemic and Paralytic Forms

After the initial infection there is a tendency for progression of symptoms, with more noticeable temperatures and signs of liver involvement at an early stage. There is considerable dispute among scientists about the exact sequence of events here and how the nervous form of the disease is caused.

Affected horses stagger before going down or may simply be found in the recumbent position. They tend to be bright and may have a good appetite but are simply unable to stand. The condition becomes progressively worse from this point as the effects of recumbency tend to cause paralysis of the limbs and ulceration of the skin if the horse is down for any length of time. The animal may be unable to pass water and constipation is not unusual.

Muscular complications are a common sequel to the systemic form of the disease and are probably linked to liver damage. Horses may be seen to move badly at work and may tend to tie up on fast exercise.

Abortion

Abortion normally occurs in the second half of pregnancy. It is a sequel to respiratory infection and occurs from two weeks to four months thereafter. However serious outbreaks can lead to abortion storms in which all normal rules are broken. In such cases there may be shortened time intervals — within days of introduction to infection — and thirty-day abortions in recently covered mares have been known.

Diagnosis: This is confirmed by virus isolation at a laboratory or by postmortem examination of the aborted foetus or dead foal.

Treatment: The course of the respiratory virus will not be affected by drugs, though it is vital that infected horses are kept warm and well nourished. Foals may have to be treated with antibiotics to control secondary invaders, but the warmth of their stables is critical to recovery; cold and draughts are not easily tolerated. Where there is liver damage, feeding may have to be adjusted to allow for a reduced protein tolerance. Horses must naturally be cut back in their work, and the value of grass as a tonic cannot be underestimated.

Recumbent horses seldom get back to their feet without help. Slings may be essential — even when these are roughly constructed, they can have the required effect. When horses are down they need to be turned several times a day to aid circulation and limit pressure ulcers. In slings, horses may tend to damage themselves and considerable padding is needed to ensure this is minimised. Fluid levels have to be maintained by administration of electrolyte solutions. Feeding should be laxative to ensure the bowel remains functional.

Aborted mares must be isolated and all contaminated material destroyed. It is obligatory to submit the aborted foetus and afterbirth for examination to a recognised laboratory.

A Code of Practice exists for this disease, details of which are available on request from the Thoroughbred Breeders' Association. It is a complex code aimed at limiting the effects of recent serious outbreaks. While it is a voluntary code it is important that it be respected and its recommendations adhered to.

Regulations are listed for actions to be taken when a mare aborts, and steps are advised to limit the spread of the disease.

Prevention: While there are vaccines available, their efficacy is questioned, and considerable money is at present being spent on research to improve the situation. Some authorities do suggest that blanket vaccination of broodmares has reduced the incidence of abortion. However the effect on the respiratory disease is not satisfactory and the exercise of using vaccine in the face of existing infection is questionable.

EHV 4, also known as EHV 1 Subtype 2

With this virus the initial respiratory disease may be more marked. However, it does not generally extend beyond the respiratory system and there is no abortion in mares.

EHV 3

This virus is the cause of pock in mares, occurring as blisters on the vulva and surrounding areas. It can be venereally transmitted to the stallion where it causes the same lesions on the penis and sheath. After healing, the damaged areas usually lose their pigment. Spread also occurs by contact through dirty tail bandages, instruments, etc.

The condition is mild and the mare usually breeds normally at the next heat period. Stallions may be out of work for a time with infection.

The incubation period is from two to six days. The vulva is painful and swollen. Healing occurs normally within 7–10 days.

This virus is also known to cause a mild respiratory disease in foals and yearlings.

In severe outbreaks of herpes virus infection it is not unusual for more than one species of virus to be isolated at the same time. This may greatly accentuate the seriousness of the problems produced.

Rotavirus Infection in Foals

This virus is the cause of an infectious scour of foals which has been a serious problem on many large stud farms in recent times. While considered to be on the wane at the moment, its importance cannot be discounted. Virtually all foals are affected, though the virus is not responsible for a high incidence of deaths. However, the condition is debilitating and the danger comes with secondary bacterial infection.

Treatment: The important factor is to limit fluid loss and restore electrolyte balance. This is done with a combination of drugs which coat the bowel and help to replace lost fluid. Milk intake is controlled while the foal is scouring. It may be necessary to fit a muzzle. Many balanced electrolyte preparations are available for oral use.

11　Parasitic Diseases

Strongyles or Redworms

This family of parasites is divided into two groups – large and small strongyles. They are the cause of continuous disease problems in horses and are occasionally responsible for death, especially in foals. While modern drugs are very effective against both groups, the condition is far from eradicated and the life-cycle of the larger strongyle makes it a continuous problem.

Life cycle: Adult worms of the large strongyles live in the intestines, the females laying eggs which are passed out in the faeces. On the pasture, or even rank bedding, a larva develops within the egg. Under conditions of moisture and warmth the larva escapes from the egg and is then capable of infecting a horse or pony. It will make its way up along the herbage where it is eaten by grazing animals. Once in the gut, larvae penetrate the wall and migrate through the arterial system where they may be responsible for forming clumps (or aneurysms). They can develop in this situation into infertile adults, or may return to the bowel where they complete their development. Some large strongyles travel via the liver and other organs. Adult large strongyles attach themselves firmly to the lining of the bowel from which they suck blood.

Immature larvae have a protective coat which allows them to survive for long periods in herbage. Under ideal conditions the egg may become infective in a week. Cold weather slows this development, thus allowing infective larvae to overwinter outside a host.

Their full life cycle, from egg laying to maturity, takes about 6–9 months.

The small strongyles differ in their cycles in that they develop in the wall of the gut from which they emerge, to grow to maturity within the lumen of the bowel. They do not suck blood and their cycle takes about six weeks from egg to adult.

Symptoms: Where large doses of larvae are taken in by worm-free animals, there may be acute illness and death within 2–3 weeks. In chronic build-up of worm burden, there is marked loss of condition, anaemia, distended stomach and a staring coat. There may be a tendency to diarrhoea. On occasion the worms may be seen in the droppings.

In heavy infestations, worm eggs will be detected in the faeces under microscopic examination. On postmortem, the wall of the bowel may contain large numbers of nodules from immature strongyles and the walls of the large arteries may contain immature worms clumped together into aneurysms.

The danger with worms in the vessel walls is their release into the arterial flow, where they may block off small vessels in which they become lodged. This may lead to serious colic. Areas of gut wall are cut off from their blood supply and die. The condition often leads to the death of the patient. This problem is most common in foals but can be seen in horses of all ages.

Diagnosis: Worms may be seen in the droppings, or eggs are found on faecal examination in the laboratory.

Treatment: The modern drug, ivermectin, is effective against both mature and larval stages of the large and small strongyles. However, there is a certain danger in killing immature larvae within arterial vessels because the dead worms may fall into the bloodstream and cause serious blockage of smaller vessels. This is not an uncommon clinical happening and should always be considered when suspicious symptoms are encountered after dosing.

Other drugs such as thiabendazole and pyrantel embonate are effective, though their efficiency against the immature stages is limited. They are still useful drugs for alternating with ivermectin in a worm elimination programme.

It is necessary to worm horses at grass regularly — every 6–8 weeks at least for intensive horse farms — as there is a constant intake of larvae. Furthermore developing worms which were not killed previously may have matured and be vulnerable.

It is possible with regular effective worming to reduce the redworm problem considerably. It is, however, still advisable to consider grazing practices and keep pastures as clean as possible. This may be done by changing horses onto fresh pasture regularly, or, alternatively, where this is not possible, cattle and sheep may be used to reduce the larval burden as strongyles do not develop in these species. Droppings may be physically removed from fields which are intensively grazed, or may be broken up so that larvae are exposed to the rays of the sun. Of course this practice also increases the spread of the larvae and so fosters their chance of being eaten.

It goes without saying that proper stable management should never allow for the development of infective larvae indoors.

The Seat Worm (Oxyuris)

This worm causes tail rubbing. This occurs because adult female seat worms attach themselves in the area of the rectum and anus. Because they are fragile, some females rupture here, releasing their eggs, and leaving a yellowish-white deposit around the anus and perineum. The eggs are sticky and adhere to stable walls and fixtures, fences and bedding. Their development is rapid, the egg turning into an infective larva in 3−5 days. The worm grows to maturity in about five months.

Suspicion of seat worm (pin worm) infestation is aroused by tail-rubbing.

Seat worms are susceptible to most of the worm drugs in use today.

White Round Worm (Ascaris)

These worms are common in the horse and donkey. They are 15−30 cm (6−12 in.) long, a yellowish white colour, pointed at one end and about as thick as a knitting-needle. They are the cause of considerable trouble in foals, where they may accumulate and virtually block the small bowel. In adult equines, they do not have the same significance.

Life cycle: The female lays her eggs in the gut and these are passed out in the droppings. Once on the pasture a larva grows within the egg and these are eaten by the next host. These eggs are very resistant to weathering. In the gut the eggs hatch and the larvae penetrate the intestinal wall and migrate throughout the internal organs to the lungs. They find their way into the windpipe, from which they are coughed up and swallowed. Returning to the gut, they grow into mature worms.

Symptoms and diagnosis: Unless present in large numbers there is little external disturbance, the diagnosis being made when the worms are seen in the droppings. Young animals with heavy infestations will be poor in condition, with staring coats and potbellies.

Treatment: This worm is susceptible to most modern worm drugs. The control of pasture contamination is best approached in the same way as with redworms.

Lungworm (Dictyocaulus)

Lungworm can be a cause of chronic coughing in horses, especially where there is direct contact with land grazed by donkeys.

Life cycle: While these are roundworms also, their life cycle is different in that the adults live in the tubes of the lungs. Eggs are laid onto the mucous covering of these tubes and are coughed or carried up to the throat. Here they join the intestinal contents and are carried out in the faeces. Eggs hatch within 48 hours of reaching the ground into a first stage larva. After another 48 hours this larva moults and becomes the second stage larva which matures to a stage which is infective in about 6–7 days. Once these larvae are eaten they migrate through the tissues to the lungs where they mature into adults.

The larval phases on the ground are inhibited by extremes of hot and cold weather. They thrive on warm humid conditions. The time lapse from larva to adult is about six weeks.

The donkey does not suffer clinically from infestation with large numbers of lungworm, a fact which makes the donkey potentially dangerous to the horse; if an infestation in a donkey is not detected, the horse is at greater risk.

Diagnosis: While the presence of a chronic dry cough may create suspicion of lungworm infestation, positive diagnosis is made when larvae are identified in faecal samples. However, a negative result is not always conclusive and it may be difficult to establish an opinion on this basis. In such cases it is best to dose with a drug such as ivermectin and observe the response.

Bots (Gastrophilus)

Most horses become infected with bots at some stage of their life, and many may carry very heavy burdens if not treated. Bots produce only one generation of larvae per year.

Life-cycle: The eggs are laid by the botfly onto the hairs of the limbs of the horse and can be seen readily as rows of small yellow objects around the knees, hocks and cannons. The horse licks the eggs from the hair, and larve from these hatch out and invade the tissues of the mouth. After about three weeks, they pass to the stomach as second stage larvae. In the stomach, these develop into third stage larvae in about 3—4 weeks. These larvae can then remain for variable periods up to 10 months before they detach and pass out in the faeces, where they eventually turn into flies. Larvae produce deep pits at the point of their attachment in the stomach, and, on occasion, they may perforate the wall and cause peritonitis.

While there has always been dispute as to whether the bot in the horse's stomach is of great clinical significance, it cannot be suggested that the animals are not better off without it.

Diagnosis: Only the presence of larvae can confirm bot infestation, and large numbers of these may be seen at times in droppings.

Treatment: Ivermectin is also effective against this worm.

Control: Eggs can be removed from the legs of horses by regular grooming with a hard brush.

Ectoparasites

Lice

Large bare patches on old and young horses are frequently caused by lice. These may be seen on the neck, flanks, shoulders and hips. The irritated skin tends to thicken from constant irritation and is susceptible to secondary infection from other organisms. Affected animals tend to lose condition rapidly. Infestation is most common in winter and spring, and reduces as the seasons get warmer.

Direct contact is the most common form of spread, but lice can be carried from one animal to another on blankets and grooming equipment, or from posts etc., on which horses scratch.

Eggs attach to the short fine hairs in areas the horse cannot reach, under the chin, for example. These hatch in 5–10 days. They feed on particles of hair and skin and some species suck blood. They mature in 21–28 days. Mature lice are about 2.5 mm (¹⁄₁₀ in.) long, and are a pale browny colour.

Diagnosis: Lice are large enough to be seen with the naked eye.

Treatment: Modern proprietary washes and powders are effective.

Mange

Sarcoptic mange affects mostly the withers, back, neck, shoulders and sides. Small lumps appear on the skin, due to the mites burrowing within it, and a yellowish liquid oozes from them. This dries, the hair falls out and a dry scaly patch is left. There is intense irritation of the skin, especially when the animal is warm, and it is constantly rubbing and biting itself. The condition is highly contagious.

Psoroptic mange is similar to sarcoptic mange except in being less irritant and is usually found at the base of the mane and tail. The mites are only differentiated under a microscope.

Chorioptic mange affects mainly the legs from the knee and hock downwards. This is seldom seen nowadays. It can be treated with various proprietary drugs on the market.

12 Disorders of the Digestive System

Diarrhoea

The causes of this condition come under several headings.

1. Infection. With infection there may or may not be a temperature, depending on the organism and the length of time the animal has been suffering.
2. Digestive disturbances — subdivided as follows:
   a. Sudden changes of food quality, as may happen where horses are moved quickly from poor to rich pasture. Illness can be very acute, as in the condition known as Colitis X. Horses may be found dead or seriously dehydrated. Professional help is needed in all cases.
   b. Changes of food variety. This may be the result of poor judgement or can happen where feed merchants are obliged to change their source of materials.
   c. High protein feeds may aggravate the bowel and cause enteritis with diarrhoea. This can occur when horses are first introduced to soya bean, etc.
   d. Overfeeding, be this accidental — as when a feedroom is broken into — or when horses are prepared too vigorously for sales, etc.
3. Heavy worm burdens.
4. Purgatives cause diarrhoea and must not be used to excess.

It should be understood that diarrhoea is always serious. The fluid loss is potentially life endangering, and the physical damage to the lining of the bowel can lead to further complications, e.g. ulceration and perforation.

Treatment: Fluid loss must be controlled and replacement therapy instituted. Antibiotics may be needed in infectious conditions and these will have to be prescribed by a qualified person.

Feeding should be simplified, the animal put on good hay alone or hay and oats if these are tolerated. In some situations the bowel needs a complete rest from food in order to repair. Foals may need to be muzzled and only allowed access to their mother under supervision.

All changes of food must be made gradually.

Constipation

This is often due to poor food quality. There may be too little roughage to stimulate the bowel, or too much to digest.

Constipation is a feature of toxic conditions which occur due to accumulation of sediment in the large bowel.

It can be a feature of the condition known as *grass sickness*, in which there are changes in parts of the nervous system.

Treatment: Where the condition is mild a laxative diet may be adequate — grass and bran mashes. However if it does not respond quickly, colic is a possible outcome and more potent therapy will be required. Epsom salts or liquid paraffin are mild in their effect and helpful in clearing the bowel.

Colic

The term is used to describe abdominal pain arising from the stomach or intestines. The horse is more susceptible to it than other animals for the following reasons:

    a. The bowel is more sensitive to pain.
    b. Gas production, often associated with introduction to fresh grass, can cause acute spasm of bowel segments.
    c. The size and dynamics of the bowel together with the athletic nature of the animal make twisting more common.

The exciting causes are:

    a. Improper digestion of food disturbs the mechanics of bowel movement.

   b. Poor quality food. Heated hay or oats will cause excess fermentation and the danger of colic from spasm or bloat.

   c. Accidental access to concentrates.

   d. Sudden changes of food.

   e. Very high protein levels can cause inflammation and ulceration of the gut.

   f. Combining too many varieties can predispose to poor digestion.

   g. Excessive drinking of cold water when hot.

   h. Ravenous feeding after heavy work.

   i. Too little exercise coupled with full working feeds.

   j. Gaseous colic is very common with sudden weather changes on lush grass.

There are several different types of colic, but, as their diagnosis requires considerable skill and experience, the various types will be dealt with collectively. The signs and symptoms at the outset are very similar, only the grade of pain is variable.

Symptoms:

   a. There is evident unease.

   b. The horse looks back at his sides and may kick at his abdomen.

   c. He may paw the ground with his forelegs.

   d. He may get up and down continually.

   e. When down, he may roll and make violent movements.

   f. The horse may attempt to pass water continually.

   g. Large amounts of wind and small amounts of droppings will be passed.

   h. The temperature is usually normal.

The rate of the pulse and the colour of the membranes help to assess if the colic is serious or not. If the pulse rate does not exceed 45–50 and the eye membranes are salmon pink, the prognosis is good.

Treatment: It is wise to summon veterinary advice as soon as any animal shows signs of colic. Many cases begin mildly and gradually become more serious. In the case of bowel spasm especially, early injection of countering drugs is essential as well as treatment to relieve pain. Horses that react violently, throwing themselves about and fretting, are in danger of physically injuring themselves. They are likely to dehydrate more quickly because of excessive sweating, and, it is often suggested, they may precipitate twisting of the bowel through their actions. Even if they do not twist the bowel, these violent reactions can reduce considerably their chances of survival.

In simple colics caused by blockage, lubricants such as liquid paraffin are helpful. The decision to administer a lubricant however, will follow internal examination. It can be dangerous to give large volumes of liquids to horses which have blockages, or twists; the condition can be made worse.

Food is withheld, as is water, though horses in pain vary in their desire for either.

The use of enemas is of doubtful value as very often the retention of faecal material in the terminal bowel is only a reflection of the problems further along.

It is important to keep the horse warm. Horses in acute pain are best kept on their feet and walking while treatment is given a chance to take effect. It is important that they are not allowed to damage themselves.

Twisted Gut

The entire bowel is coated by a thin layer of tissue called the peritoneum. This layer combines with the mesentery which, more or less, suspends the whole mass from the roof of the abdomen. Within these confines, there is certain scope for movement. A section of the small intestine called the *ileum* is most commonly twisted because it has a relatively long mesentery, but any part of the gut can be involved.

Within a twisted segment there is often an inclination for gas to accumulate. Also blood supply is impeded, perhaps causing tissues to die. Pain becomes acute.

While the prognosis is poor, extremely good surgical work is done on the condition today. Even if the percentage of animals surviving is not high, if the level of pain can be controlled to enable a strong animal to be transported to an equipped surgery, the risk is worthwhile. No one likes to see a horse suffer, however, and in hopeless cases a decision has to made on humane grounds.

Symptoms: In the early stages, symptoms may not be easy to distinguish, but:

a. The pulse is substantially increased and thready in nature.
b. There is a tendency to profuse, patchy sweating.
c. The level of pain varies, but can become so great as to make the animal extremely violent.
d. The eye membranes become injected, i.e. a deep red colour.
e. The temperature may rise to 104 or 105, but this is variable.
f. There may be audible sounds from the bowel.
g. Breathing is accelerated during spasms of pain.
h. On rectal examination, the bowel may cling to the hand. The terminal bowel will be relatively empty. Pain will be acute as the hand reaches forward from the pelvis into the abdomen.

In many cases of colic the horse may squat as if trying to pass urine, and, in some cases, the animal will continually pass small quantities. It will be found as the condition is relieved that these symptoms pass off.

Choking

This is a blockage of the oesophagus, somewhere between the throat and the stomach. It can be caused by an object such as an apple or a potato, a large piece of root, even a mass of hay or dry food bolted down by a greedy feeder.

The symptoms are salivation, frequent attempts at swallowing, and gurgling sounds. At intervals the head may be drawn into the chest, the muscles of the neck are flexed to force the food down, then the head is stretched out again. If one stands on the near side and observes the neck along the jugular groove, an upward wave of movement can be seen. The animal salivates and champs his jaws. The horse may be helped by light massage down the jugular groove on the near side.

If the condition is not quickly resolved expert advice should be sought.

The Teeth

For efficient working of the digestive system each compartment must fulfil its separate purpose. In the mouth, food must be properly chewed, but irregularities of the teeth may prevent it. The molar teeth develop sharp edges with normal wear and these are found on the cheek side of the upper row and on the tongue side of the lower row. It happens because of the basic construction of the teeth and the way in which food is ground between them. These sharp edges may cut into the soft tissues to either side of them, thus causing pain for the animal when he eats.

Symptoms:

      a. Quidding — partly chewed food may fall from the mouth in wet clumps.

      b. The head may be held to one side and the movement of the jaws be cautious and restricted.

      c. The damage to the soft tissues can be seen and the sharp edges felt — with care.

Treatment: The edges are removed with a tooth rasp. To facilitate the exercise and avoid damage to the tongue, a gag can be inserted to open the mouth. While excessive rasping is unwise, some edges may need firm pressure.

Sloppy food should be given to horses with sore mouths for a few days to allow for recovery.

Molar teeth may be *broken* through injury; perhaps from a kick. There will be pain when the animal is eating or being ridden, especially if the bit causes pressure on the broken tooth. Diagnosis may require x-rays, and the damaged tooth may have to be surgically removed.

Lampas (a swelling of the mucous membrane of the hard palate) is not recognised as a clinical condition today.

13 Diseases of the Respiratory System

These are among the most common problems of racing and competing horses today. Environmental factors have a major part to play in precipitating them. It is a complex subject which should be given a great deal of thought by horse owners. The health of the respiratory system is influenced by ventilation, insulation, temperature changes and factors such as bedding and hay quality, not forgetting the design and construction of buildings. We have mentioned previously the defence mechanisms which are constantly fighting off infection of the respiratory system. Any factor which reduces the efficiency of these will foster the development of disease.

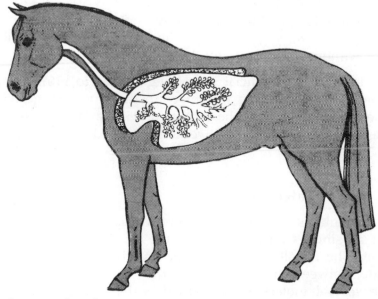

Lungs and trachea

Coughing

Coughing results from irritation of the tissues of the throat and is common in inflammatory conditions of this area.

    a. Coughing may result from infection, though many throat infections are not marked by coughing.
    b. It can reflect a deeper source. Coughing is not uncommon in infections and allergies affecting the lung tissues.
    c. It can result from worm infestations.
    d. It can follow congestion of the lungs where the primary problem is in the circulatory system.
    e. It is a response to mechanical suffocation by inhaled dirt.

Treatment:

    a. If there is bacterial infection, antibiotics may be needed to offset it.
    b. Drugs which stimulate respiratory secretions help to bring trapped material to the nostrils. Even inhalations and simple applications like Vick have their use.
    c. Where coughing is due to worms the horse will need to be treated for these.
    d. Chronic coughing frequently reflects unsuitable stabling. Often, moving the animal to better conditions will stop it without the use of any drugs.

While exercise is beneficial in helping horses to bring up accumulated foreign material from the lower respiratory passages, it should never be too vigorous until the condition is in hand. If horses suffering from respiratory infections are worked too hard, it will only prolong the problem.

Sinus Infection

The skull contains several cavities known as sinuses. There are four pairs of air-sinuses on each side of the head and they all intercommunicate. The maxillary sinuses over the cheek teeth are divided on each side, between the fourth and fifth molars, into two halves. The roots of several molars are contained within them. The sinuses are positioned above the nasal passages and onto the front of the face.

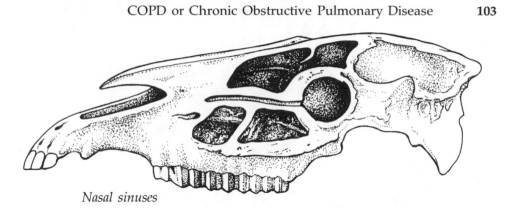

Nasal sinuses

Sinus infection may occur as a result of extension upwards from damaged teeth, though it is far more common as a complication of respiratory conditions, with the source of infection entering the air spaces through small openings in the nasal passages.

Symptoms: Nasal discharge is a common sign, though, in some cases, the sinus may be closed and pus contained within it. Depending on the level of infection, discharges may also contain blood. The glands of the head are not swollen as a result of sinus infection and there is no sound to be heard on normal breathing. Horses exercised with inflamed sinuses, however, may make some inspiratory noise. In severe cases of infection, there is distortion of the bones of the face.

Diagnosis: The discharge is often one-sided. Pain may be detected on palpation over the infected area.

Treatment: Infected sinuses are frequently opened by surgery. Antibiotics can be of help, as can drugs which help the sinuses to drain naturally.

COPD or Chronic Obstructive Pulmonary Disease

This condition, also known as 'heaves', or 'broken wind', is an allergy to the spores of fungi and moulds which are commonly found in dusty hay and straw. It is a disease of horses over five years, though often seen in younger animals. It is characterised by a chronic cough, by laboured exhalation, nasal discharge, and a low exercise tolerance.

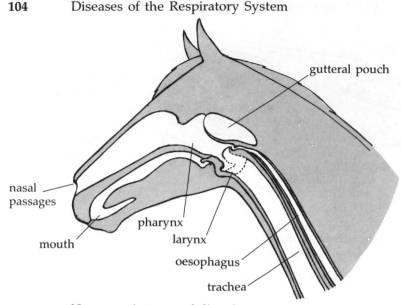

Upper respiratory and digestive passages

COPD is a disease of the indoor horse, as the symptoms are generally reduced or absent when the animal is at grass. The spores that cause it can saturate dust in stables and be presented to susceptible animals when the bedding or hay is shaken up and even when dust on walls and ceiling is agitated by coughing. The disease can lead to emphysema, which is marked by wheezing, increased breathing rate, and by difficulty in taking breath. The wall of the stomach lifts with each inhalation and there is a marked line — called the heave line — along the bottom of the ribs and abdomen. A double movement marks exhalation, due to contraction of the stomach muscles in an attempt to empty the lungs of air.

There are all grades of this condition, varying from the mild to the suffocating. Many horses live with the condition and perform perfectly useful duties. Also, with the advent of several modern drugs, the influence of COPD has been brought under greater control.

Symptoms: First the horse will suffer from a reduced exercise tolerance. In a racehorse, this will show up as poor performance at work and racing. Coughing may not be noticed, although the resting respiratory rate will be increased and a watery nasal discharge may be seen.

As the condition advances, breathing becomes more laboured and the performance of the animal suffers accordingly. The membranes of the nose and eye become notably congested, and coughing — a deep abdominal cough — may become persistent. Loud wheezing sounds are heard from the lungs and the efforts to expel inhaled air are marked.

Diagnosis: The condition is distinguished from other respiratory conditions which increase the breathing rate. There is no temperature, no infectious discharge, and the animal is often bright and in good condition despite his very poor exercise tolerance.

Treatment: The drug clenbuterol is useful in controlling the symptoms. Its effect is to relieve spasm of the lungs and help the removal of foreign materials. Many other useful drugs are also available, e.g. sodium cromoglycate which is given by inhalation, mainly as a preventive.

Control: Management of COPD horses is a matter of prime importance.

- a. They must be kept in an atmosphere free of dust.
- b. Attention must be paid to the quality of hay fed. It must be well made, dust-free and preferably damped. Some horses with COPD can tolerate no hay and they may then be fed exclusively on grass or haylage.
- c. Straw bedding should be replaced by shavings or paper.
- d. The stable must be clean and dust-free.
- e. If other horses in an open building are not kept in the same manner they will serve to promote the condition by stirring allergens into the atmosphere.
- f. A great deal is written about ventilation for horses suffering from COPD. While it has to be appreciated that any animal having difficulty getting oxygen needs plenty of air, draughty conditions inhibit the natural defences of the respiratory system. It is not difficult to marry the two needs so that a horse is adequately ventilated and still warm.
- g. COPD is life-lasting, and animals who suffer with it need to be protected from its effects continually. However, modern therapies allow many horses to live full competitive lives in spite of it.

Pneumonia

The term is used to describe infection of the lungs. This is normally bacterial, though often secondary in nature. Viral pneumonia is called *pneumonitis*, and is generally not as damaging to lung tissue cells. However, it opens the door to bacterial infections which are more likely to kill the animal.

Any problem which lowers infection resistance may lead to pneumonia. Thus a combination of exposure, poor feeding and bad stabling may be the cause. It may occur when food goes the wrong way, or after worm infestations when there has been migration of larvae through the lungs.

Symptoms: A significant rise in temperature occurs at an early stage, accompanied by an increase in respiratory rate and pulse. The animal may sweat slightly or be seen to shiver. There may or may not be a cough. The nostrils are dilated and if there is associated pleurisy – which is an extension of the infection onto the linings of the chest cavity – there is marked pain on breathing.

Diagnosis: Parts of the lung become consolidated with pneumonia. A veterinary surgeon can detect this on examination.

Treatment: Antibiotics are indicated early, and the response is likely to be good. The horse must be kept warm and out of draughts. The atmosphere must be clean and healthy so that oxygen is readily available, because the condition means that there is reduced lung space for gas exchange.

The prognosis with pneumonia today is good. The animal will need professional attendance, but may make a complete recovery in a matter of days in response to effective treatment.

Whistling and Roaring

These conditons are dealt with under one heading since the changes involved are similar and differ only in degree. The cause is a change in the structures of the larynx.

The names are self-explanatory and have been coined to describe

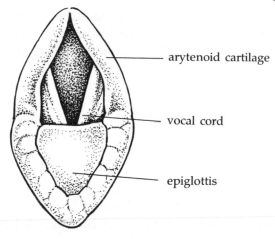

arytenoid cartilage

vocal cord

epiglottis

The larynx of the horse

the noises made by affected horses. Their significance can be best appreciated with some knowledge of the anatomy of the organ involved.

The larynx is a hollow, rigid structure whose walls are made up of cartilages united through joints and ligaments, lined on the inside by a continuation of the mucous membrane of the throat and windpipe. This membrane is raised to form a pair of vocal cords each of which enfolds the underlying vocal ligament. During inhalation the vocal cords are closed, to allow free access of air to the lungs. Both relax on expiration.

The movements of the larynx are controlled by a number of small muscles which are innervated by a slender nerve, named the recurrent laryngeal, on either side of the neck. Each of these nerves follows a tortuous path. At the base of the neck on the right side the nerve winds round a small artery and then runs back up the jugular groove along with the common carotid artery to the larynx. The left nerve passes back even further into the chest before it winds round the large main artery at the base of the heart and then follows the same course as the right nerve up the neck.

As roaring and whistling are due to partial paralysis of the left vocal cord, and this is related to damage in the left nerve, various theories abound as to how this happens. The most popular belief is that the damage is physical due to stretching of the nerve as it passes round the artery at the base of the heart. This has never been fully proven. There is a recognised genetic link and it is strongly advised that horses suffering from the problem should not be bred from. While there is also a suggestion that the condition may follow infection, this has never been established. Many horses make a noise after infection which passes off again.

Right-sided paralysis is infrequent; up to 90 per cent of cases involve the left cord.

As the paralysis develops, the cord loses its capacity to withdraw fully as air is inspired. This then forms a partial obstruction to the flow and causes the abnormal sounds heard. To begin with, only a slight noise may be heard. This is described as a whistle, and is heard in a cantering horse when all four legs are off the ground and he is filling his lungs with air. As the condition progresses, the noise becomes more pronounced and deeper and is then described as roaring. A horse does not become a roarer first and a whistler later.

A slight whistle may not interfere significantly with performance, but the more advanced condition inhibits air flow to the lungs and causes the animal to become short of breath at faster gaits.

Other problems which may obscure the condition are:

    a. Paralysis of the soft palate. In this condition the soft palate is flaccid and able to create turbulent noises in the path of incoming air.

    b. Bridle noises. These occur when the horse is ridden or lunged with its head in a flexed position. It is important the horse be allowed to breathe normally. The same may occur with dropped nosebands which can inhibit the nostrils, or other faults associated with bridle and bit.

    c. Infections in the region of the pharynx, larynx, nasal passages and lungs. Noises arising in this way often pass off again.

    d. Infection of glands and related discharges — to which the same applies as for c.

    e. Presenting horses in a fat and unfit condition to be examined. Before any horse is subjected to a test for his wind it is vital that he has been lunged or ridden for an adequate time in the days prior to the examination. He should be capable of doing what exercise is required easily and without effort or resentment. Horses taken straight out of a field are placed under a strain and may fail to satisfy their examiner only because it

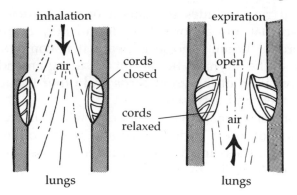

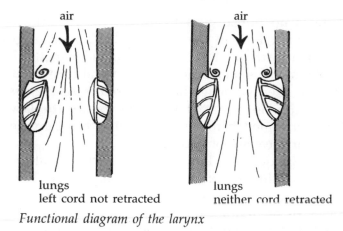

Functional diagram of the larynx

is not possible to subject them to an adequate exercise test.

f. Horses which are high-blowers make a characteristic noise when ridden. It is a noise that comes as air rushes into the false nostril and is in no way abnormal.

g. Noises which occur as the animal is exhaling are not usually significant.

Diagnosis: The condition is diagnosed through physical examination at rest and at exercise, after which special tests may be undertaken. Examination of the wind is most frequently carried out as part of a general examination for soundness. However, in such a case, if an abnormal noise is heard, the animal would usually fail the test and no further examination would be undertaken.

The examination at rest includes evaluation of the cardiac and respiratory systems, so that any abnormalities found may be related to noises heard at exercise. When a noise is heard it is common for an internal examination of the larynx to be carried out using an endoscope. This way the true condition of the vocal cords and other tissues in the area can be directly seen and assessed.

It needs to be appreciated that there are horses which make inspiratory noises which do not affect performance and which often tend to become less marked as fitness increases. An objective assessment has to be made of the horse's ability to perform as well as consideration of any lesions found.

Treatment: There is no nonsurgical treatment for the true condition which is marked by paralysis of the vocal cord. Various surgical operations are undertaken with great frequency. The older method involves the stripping of the mucous membranes of the vocal cords and is called a Hobday operation, after the man who pioneered it. As the tissues heal the cord is drawn into close contact with the wall of the larynx. This operation, when performed before the condition has become too advanced, enjoys a fair measure of success.

Other surgical techniques, including the tie-back operation, involve restoring the shape of the larynx from outside its lumen. The mucous membrane of the vocal cord is normally stripped as well.

There is no way of preventing the condition, although its incidence might be reduced if steps were taken to stop the breeding of affected animals. In many countries stallions at stud are not licensed if suffering from this condition. However, unfortunately, this stipulation does not apply to Thoroughbred breeding.

The condition, it has to be said, is mainly one of larger horses and is uncommon in those under 16 hh.

14 Conditions Relating to the Circulatory System

Heart Disease

The diagnosis of heart conditions is a very specialised exercise which is best left exclusively in the hands of professionals. This is true even when an owner suspects the presence of a problem. The study of the heart is complex, and understanding its normal variations involves a great deal of learning. Many professionals themselves find the subject too complex and leave it to specialists. This indicates how little chance lay people have of correctly assessing heart conditions in the horse.

As described in circulation of the blood, the return flow to the heart passes into the two atria, right and left, and when both are full the walls contract to force the blood into the right and left ventricles. Between each atrium and its corresponding ventricle there is a valve. When open, this permits blood flow from atrium to ventricle. Once the ventricle is full the valves close with a sound which is audible with a stethoscope. The ventricle then contracts, forcing blood into the lungs and through the main arteries of the body. There are two valves between the ventricles and the large vessels leaving them. The pulmonary valve is in the artery leading to the lungs; the aortic valve is in the artery conveying blood to the body generally. At the end of contraction, when the ventricles are empty and the walls relaxed, these two valves close with another audible sound. Two basic sounds can therefore be heard in one heart cycle which differ in tone. These are commonly described by the words *lubb-dup*. The longer, deeper *lubb* sound is related to the atrioventricular valves; *dup* is a short sound corresponding to the closure of the pulmonary and aortic valves.

Deviations from these heart sounds occur normally. In the athletic animal, when the heart is slowed to its resting rate, four heart sounds may be heard, and this is not abnormal. Beats may be dropped for a variety of reasons and this is not always a sign of disease. Toxins will cause this as will certain drugs and feed supplements. A distinction between what is acceptable and what is not should be made by an experienced veterinary surgeon.

It is occasionally suggested that *dropped beats* at rest indicate added reserve in a fit animal. This is a dangerous assumption to make as the condition may be pathological. Even where the condition is marked, however, a horse may be functionally normal − as long as the heart works efficiently at exercise. Many horses have abnormal resting heart patterns and are still sound.

Murmurs are sounds which are not present in normal heart contraction. However this does not mean they all indicate disease. Many murmurs are not clinically significant. They are taken into account as they relate to the practical working of the organ when the animal is subjected to exercise. Many good horses which have been condemned as unsound from murmurs have become winners of the country's top races.

Epistaxis

This is a term used to describe bleeding from the nostrils. It is commonly associated with exercise, and recent suggestions are made that a large percentage of race horses have some degree of bleeding during races, even where there is no apparent external sign of it.

There are numerous points in the respiratory system from which bleeding can occur. While any bleeding indicates damage to a vessel, the relationship with prior infection is often marked. Lesions caused by infection may erode the walls of small blood vessels and weaken them. The pressure of exercise will then lead to breakdown and bleeding. At postmortem, bleeding is often found to have occurred deep in the tissues of the lungs.

Spontaneous nasal bleeding from horses not at exercise can vary from light to profuse. Sometimes infection of the gutteral pouch − which runs between the pharynx and the ear − is the cause. Because this pouch overlies the large vessels in the angle behind the head, bleeding can be serious and even cause death.

Diagnosis: The animal showing signs of nasal bleeding is examined by endoscope and x-rays, if thought necessary, to locate the area of damage.

Treatment: While there are many proprietary drugs being sold as cures or preventives for this condition, their influence is mixed. It is important to locate the lesion and treat any infection which may exist. The influence of environmental factors is well recognised and there is good reason to believe that horses which have bled recover better when turned out to grass.

Lasix is used for racehorses with this condition — this is allowed in several states in the U.S.A. It is a diuretic, and its effect may result from the reduction of blood volume. There is some dispute as to the drug's performance-enhancing properties, and it has no effect on the longterm course of the disease.

The nostril of a bleeding animal should never be plugged. Immediate care should include keeping him quiet and warm, and feeding with sloppy feeds. The bleeding will usually stop spontaneously. If not, professional help is required.

The gutteral pouches can be 'scoped' and infections in them treated directly.

Filling of the Legs

While the legs of horses confined to their boxes are likely to fill, i.e. swell, through lack of exercise, the condition is more commonly related to toxic conditions stemming from the bowel. In these cases, laxatives or purgatives may be needed to relieve the symptoms. The horse is then returned to a simple diet of hay and small quantities of oats.

All horses which remain on hard feed for any length of time need a purgative at least once annually. This helps clear accumulated dirt from the bowel and is an aid to digestion in the longterm.

Some horse's legs fill when fed on heavy concentrate diets, and the only rational answer is to cut back or change the feed.

Most legs fill after injuries and this distinct type of filling is associated with wounds and grazes. They take longer to disappear, but need not always keep the animal out of work.

Lymphangitis

The lymphatic system has been described in an earlier chapter. It exists on the venous side of the circulation and carries lymph into the venous system and liver from the extremities and bowel. Along the course of these vessels the lymph glands are set, their purpose is to filter off foreign material and prevent it from getting deeper into the body.

The term lymphangitis mainly applies to a condition marked by extensive filling of one hind leg. It occurs in housed animals on hard feed.

Symptoms: The swelling is much greater than normal and the skin may even weep in severe cases. There is usually localised pain on the course of leg vessels. The animal may sweat and have a raised temperature. Lameness of the affected limb is marked.

Diagnosis: This is based on the nature and size of the swelling. Do not confuse with physical injuries.

Treatment: Antihistamine and anti-inflammatory drugs are used to control the tissue reactions which lead to the condition. In some cases the response is quick. Laxative diets and purgatives may help, as may diuretics. It is important to encourage the animal to use the affected leg in order to assist circulation.

The affected limb may retain permanent signs and each ensuing episode — recurring incidents are normal — may leave the leg a little larger. Horses which have suffered one attack should be exercised regularly and lightly lunged on rest days.

Azoturia, tying-up, etc.

This complex, known by a variety of names today, is a disease of nutrition, circulation and the muscular system. It was once known as Monday Morning Disease, because it was common in working horses which had been rested on Sundays on full rations. It has many grades, hence the names vary, and all are marked by muscular involvement of some degree.

Scientific literature divides the problem into different conditions. Clinically they are so closely related that the exercise is unnecessary here.

Symptoms: The animal may be short-striding on leaving his stable. This may progress — or it can occur spontaneously — to a point where he stiffens completely and is unable to move. Profuse sweating and blowing occurs in acute azoturia. Muscles of the loins and quarters stiffen and become painful to touch. The urine may darken to a deep brown or bloody colour. There may be a rise in temperature.

Diagnosis: This is based on the symptoms and history of the animal. Blood tests taken at the time will show substantial rises in some enzyme levels. Signs of muscle damage are visible on gross examination however, and the animal has to be treated at once to relieve pain and other symptoms.

Treatment: In mild attacks the animal should be walked gently back to his stable or transport. Some horses cannot be moved except in a box or trailer.

Pain killers may be necessary to aid recovery and relieve the acute effects on afflicted muscle. Other drugs will neutralise symptoms, and judicious physiotherapy will help return the animal to work within days.

The causes of this condition have become more complex with the passage of time and it is advisable to seek professional advice where it is recurrent.

Horses susceptible to azoturia should have their diet reduced when rested and should be warmed up gradually before hard work.

The Blood

Anaemia

In anaemia there is a reduction in the oxygen-carrying capacity of the blood. This is due to a deficiency of red cells, or to an inability of RBCs to carry adequate oxygen.

For performing horses, this is a serious limitation as it restricts the animals' capacity to work.

Causes:

    a. Blood loss through haemorrhage.
    b. Severe worm burdens.
    c. Deficiencies of the food elements vital to red blood cell formation, e.g. iron, vitamin B12, folic acid, etc.

d. Damage to the organs responsible for red cell generation; the liver, and bone marrow.
e. Excessive breakdown of red cells, e.g. in infection.

Diagnosis: The condition is not clinically recognised unless the loss is marked, when the membranes of the body appear pale and bleached, and the animal may be poor in condition and have breathing problems at light exercise.

Less-marked stages are diagnosed professionally and will be confirmed by blood testing, when the figures for total red cells, haemoglobin level and packed cell volume will be below accepted levels.

It should be appreciated that levels which are consistent with outward normality may not allow a racehorse to run to his form. Very small percentage differences affect the athlete.

Treatment: This involves treating the specific cause and replacing any items missing from the diet. Drugs called haematinics stimulate the production of red cells.

Dehydration

As the name implies, this term represents a loss of fluid from the body. It can mean a loss from any of the three main fluid compartments, namely, the blood, extracellular fluid and intracellular fluid. All these compartments are in a state of dynamic equilibrium, so they compensate for each other across the various membranes that divide them. Inevitably, the fluid within cells cannot be significantly removed without endangering the life of the whole animal, so the other compartments have to protect the cells at their own cost.

Causes:

a. Excessive sweating is the most common reason for dehydration, especially if the lost electrolytes are not replaced.
b. As a result of virus or bacterial infections.
c. From inadequate water intake.
d. From excessive water loss, e.g. in diarrhoea and urinary conditions.

e. In conditions of acute pain such as colic.
f. In shock, after accidents or surgery.
g. During transportation on long journeys.

Symptoms: Gross dehydration is marked by lethargy, dry skin and reduced exercise tolerance. Because the blood has less of its fluid element, it thickens, thus making it harder for the heart to pump it through the circulation.

If the skin of a dehydrated horse is pinched, the fold of skin is delayed in returning to its normal position.

In severe dehydration the animal will die unless the lost fluid is replaced.

Diagnosis: Must be formed from knowledge of the horse and any excess fluid loss. Confirmation on blood-testing shows increased packed cell volume.

Treatment: While the treatment of clinical dehydration is a matter for the professional and may require fluid replacement by intravenous means, the normal fluid level of competing or working horses is the responsibility of the individual horseman.

There are many proprietary sources of electrolytes for oral use available. It is important that horses receive an available and balanced source — after strenuous exercise, where there has been extensive sweating, or as a routine at least once a week while in work.

15   Conditions of the Eye

Because of the delicate nature of the tissues of the eye, and the serious results which can follow improper treatment, only the more basic conditions will be considered here.

Injury

Bruising of the eyelids and the bones forming the socket may occur accidentally. The eyelids become swollen and there is a profuse release of tears. As long as the eyeball is not damaged, the injury will respond to bathing. Pain-killers or anti-inflammatory drugs may be needed in some cases.

If the lids are torn they will need to be stitched in order to retain their shape. Their function is to protect the eyeball and help clear out foreign matter by regular movement. If a tear is not stitched the integrity of the lids is broken and foreign material can gain access to the eye.

Conjunctivitis

This term is used to denote inflammation of the membrane covering the inside of the eyelids, known as the conjunctiva. It may result from injury, irritation from dust etc., from a foreign object, or as a complication of systemic infection. Generally it is not in itself serious but it may lead to keratitis.

Treatment: Any foreign body present should be removed at once and the eye irrigated with warm water. If the case is a simple inflammation, without infection, flushing with a bland proprietary solution should help. Epsom salts may be used at a strength of one teaspoon to one pint of boiled water.

All water used to bathe eyes should have been boiled before use, to sterilise it and remove irritant deposits.

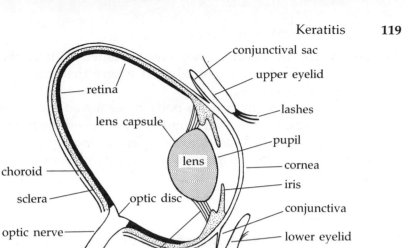

Cross section of eye

Should infection be present, as evidenced by a thick discharge, treatment will need to incorporate an antibiotic.

If conjunctivitis is a complication of some general disease, the underlying cause will have to be treated.

Keratitis

This is the term used to describe inflammation of the membrane forming the front of the eyeball, known as the cornea. It may result from direct injury, following infection of the conjunctiva, or from a foreign object.

Symptoms: Unlike other tissue which becomes red when inflamed, the cornea becomes bluey-white. This is due to the fact that the cornea is not supplied with blood vessels, since these would reduce the light entering the eye. The blueish colour reflects extensive cell damage.

Early symptoms will be marked by pain. The eyelids tend to be held closed and the eye may water profusely. If there is ulceration of the cornea, this needs professional treatment.

Diagnosis: The predominant sign is the blue discolouration of the front of the eye.

Treatment: Many modern drugs have specific use in eye conditions, but considerable damage may be done if not correctly applied. Drugs containing anti-inflammatory agents such as cortisone are used to limit damage to delicate tissues. They are combined with antibiotics where infection is a risk, but are not advised where their effect will dampen essential repair processes.

It is essential that any foreign body be removed. Small objects, such as oat husks, can become surrounded by a false membrane of opaque material. The object will be detectable in the membrane's centre.

If a wound or ulcer is present on the cornea, expert advice must be sought.

Cataract

To appreciate this condition, refer to the diagram of the eye at the beginning of the chapter. The lens is an egg-shaped structure made of clear material, contained within an outer membrane. Cataract is an opacity of the lens, of varying degrees. It may result from injury, infection, nutrition, or can be hereditary. It may result from systemic conditions as well as purely local influences. A cataract can include the whole of the lens or only part of it, and can involve one or both eyes.

Cataract is often a progressive condition and its influence on sight will vary from partial interference to total blindness. As the condition is not easily seen on gross examination, an ophthalmoscope is required for full inspection. This is one of the many reasons why horses are best subjected to full soundness examination on purchase.

Treatment for this condition today is generally surgical, although many horses live out a useful life despite diminishing sight.

Blindness

This may be caused by many things. It may be congenital or acquired, temporary or permanent, partial or complete. If it is only partial or affecting one eye, it will not be easy to detect at once.

While a rider will easily know if a horse is totally blind, any partial loss of sight is not so easy to detect. Many good horses will successfully jump and race with only one eye, or with partial blindness in one or both. Detection of these conditions is subject to examination with an ophthalmoscope.

Obviously it is important to know early about any reduction of eyesight, even if nothing can be done to correct the problem. The knowledge could well save a rider's life.

16　Conditions of the Skin

Warts

Warts, also called papillomas, are most commonly seen about the nose and lips of horses. They are caused by a virus and the disease is self-limiting in so much as the warts usually disappear within a matter of months of appearing. They leave no scar and normally do not require surgical removal. They have an incubation period of 2−3 months from time of contact to the appearance of a growth. In cases that do not recover, a vaccine may be produced from wart material at competent laboratories. However the results of such vaccines are not always satisfactory.

Sarcoids

These are skin tumours which appear on the insides of the hind legs, the sheath and udder, on the abdomen and flank, the lower part of the chest, and less often on the head and shoulders. They are firm and fibrous to the touch and vary in size from that of a wart to 10 cm across, or more. They are normally benign growths but can become malignant.

Where a sarcoid is in a position that is likely to cause problems, e.g. under the girth or saddle, or on the udder of a broodmare, it may be necessary to remove it. If it is of manageable size and has a neck to it − as opposed to being flush against the skin − a ligature, or rubber band may be used to stop its blood supply, after which it will fall off in about 10 days. However many instances are known where removal is followed by regrowth.

Modern surgical techniques involve cauterisation and are successful in dealing with the problem.

Melanoma

This is the common skin growth seen in grey horses. Again they may be benign or malignant. They tend to develop with age and are unusual in horses under five or six years. As they get older, a high percentage of grey horses are affected.

These tumours can grow on any part of the body, but are most common in the region of the perinaeum. They can be multiple, firm to handle and vary in size up to several inches. Bigger growths may have ulcers on their surface.

While surgery is performed if the growth is causing a distinct problem, they tend to regrow and continue developing. Most benign growths on grey animals are best left alone.

Warbles

The horse is not a natural host for the larva of the warble fly, and the incidence of its appearance has greatly reduced with the significant lowering of infestation in cattle. However when a warble is found under the saddle area of a ridden horse it is best to set the saddle off the nodule. This is best done by the use of a foam pad, through which a hole is cut so that the saddle does not bear on the affected area. If it is a warble, the larva will emerge in time and the condition will be resolved. Any efforts to remove it could lead to rupture of the larva with a consequent local reaction which may last for months.

The condition is so uncommon nowadays that it is unlikely to be seen in many horses. Most lesions which are confused with warbles turn out to be painful galls from saddle or tack.

Galls

The term is used to describe pressure sores which result from rubbing by the saddle or girth. They vary from slight abrasions to very painful swellings. In areas overlying bone, bursitis may occur, and this can be difficult to clear up.

The rational approach to galls is to remove the cause. If they are the result of badly fitting tack, then the remedy is self-evident. When it is important to keep the animal in exercise, no weight must be borne by the affected part. The alternative is to rest the animal until the condition has resolved itself.

Where there is bursitis, more precise local treatment may be necessary. Very often, ultrasound or laser therapy will relieve the pain. However it is vital to keep weight off damaged parts, even if this means the rider has to correct faulty riding techniques.

Cracked Heels, Grease and Mud Fever

These conditions all represent dermatitis at the back of the pastern and legs, even to as high as the knee or hock. They commonly involve more than one leg. They are caused by exposure to damp and dirt, poor stable hygiene, and to improper management of horses after exercise in wet conditions. They are more common in unpigmented legs.

They vary from mild surface irritations to severe inflammation with cracking of the skin and outpouring of serous fluid. The horse may be lame. Secondary bacterial infection is a common complication.

This heading includes the conditions referred to as *mallenders* and *sallenders*, (both are forms of dermatitis), except these occur at the back of the knee and the front of the hock respectively.

The first priority is to remove the cause. If stable management has allowed its development, it must be corrected.

The habit of hosing dirt from the legs of exercised horses is preferable to washing by hand, in which case fine dirt may be rubbed into the skin. The legs should ideally be dried off after hosing. A mild ointment such as vaseline can be used as a preventive, especially on unpigmented areas.

Where the condition exists, mild astringent lotions are used. In more severe cases, antibiotic ointments combined with anti-inflammatory drugs may be required. Where there is secondary bacterial infection, antibiotics by parenteral injection may be necessary.

Sweet Itch

This condition is troublesome to ponies particularly, though it is common in horses of all ages. It is caused by an allergy to the saliva of biting flies and seen in spring and summer in animals kept at grass.

The lesions are most commonly confined to the mane and tail and usually involve thickening of the skin with varying degrees of irritation. Affected parts are usually scratched bare.

Efforts to save the animal from contact with the fly can be of help. All sorts of techniques are used with a wide variety of success. Antifly dressings are applied to the part, and fly-repellant tabs are available for attachment to headcollars. Some owners keep affected animals in by day and out at night, when the flies are least active.

Local treatment of affected areas may involve the use of lotions and drugs which relieve the symptoms, though there is a serious likelyhood of the condition recurring.

17 Lameness

Today lameness is a specialised field involving a great deal of study and observation.

While the diagnosis of acute conditions may at times be relatively uncomplicated — because the affected leg is evident, and a distinct swelling present — determining the significance, and treatment, may involve complex considerations in order to restore full use of the limb. Diagnosis of less-serious lameness is much more difficult and it takes not only training but experience to pinpoint deep-seated causes.

Where lameness is not pronounced, the following hints may be of value:

   a. Examine the horse in his stall paying particular attention to how he is bearing weight on his limbs and whether he is pointing any one of them.

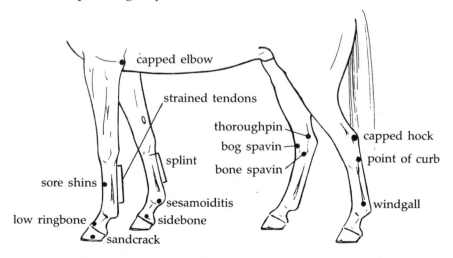

Some common sites of lameness

124

b. Take him out and observe from every angle while he is held square on a level surface. Look particularly for muscle wastage and see if the animal is standing level behind.

c. Have the horse walked away from you and back towards you, taking special note if lameness is accentuated on the turn.

d. Have the horse trotted away from you and back towards you, watching the movement of the head in relation to the place-ment of the feet on the ground. When the horse is trotting towards you, he will lift his head as the affected limb strikes the ground, if lameness is in a foreleg; the head will drop when the sound limb hits the ground. When trotting away, the sound hip drops as the same limb strikes the ground, and the head rises. The hip of the affected side rises when the limb bears weight, and the head drops.

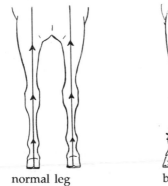

normal leg

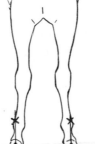

base wide, toe out

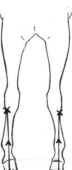

base wide, toe in

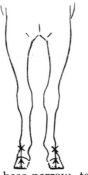

base narrow, toe out

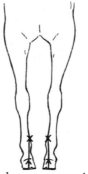

base narrow, toe in

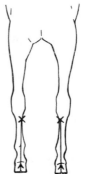

normal base, toe in

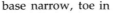

Paths of concussion

It is important to distinguish between *supporting leg lameness* — when the pain is felt as the foot meets the ground — and *swinging leg lameness* — when the pain occurs as the limb is in motion. In the latter, the movement of the head is not significant but the stride of the affected limb is shortened.

Having decided which limb is affected, certain features of movement will assist location of the injured area.

Shoulder

When in motion, the affected limb is not extended as far forward as the sound limb. The toe may be dragged and the neck muscles are more obviously used to assist forward movement of the limb. At rest the limb may be flexed with the toe resting on the ground.

Elbow

In movement, weight is taken first by the toe with the knee slightly flexed. At rest, the elbow may be dropped and the knee and fetlock flexed.

Knee

In lameness relating to the knee joint, the limb is held flexed at rest, with the knee itself bearing little weight. Lameness is usually acute at the trot.

Cannon

Splint — the affected limb may be carried further out from the body than its fellow.
Sore Shins — a short choppy step may be accompanied by the horse standing over at the knee.

Pastern

Ringbone — the stride is shortened and the lameness is accentuated on turning.

Foot

Corn — the horse will try to relieve pressure on the affected part.
Navicular disease — short stride with marked, intermittent lameness.

Hip

There is shortening of the stride with the toe striking the ground first.
The haunch on the affected side is lifted noticeably.

Stifle

The stride is shortened and the toe inclined laterally. At rest the joint is
flexed.

Hock

Improper extension of the affected leg and dragging of the toe when
moving.

All of the above are only a guide and it must be appreciated that,
with the limbs of the horse, there is a great deal of counter-action
between joints; this influences the way the limb is moved and relaxed.
If, for example, the hock is flexed, the stifle and fetlock are also flexed.
This is because of the existence of a reciprocal apparatus in the hind
leg.

Lameness relating to problems in the back is marked by changes of
stride pattern which may affect more than one leg.

The following are specific types of lameness.

Shoulder Lameness

While shoulder lameness — that is lameness originating in the scapulo-
humeral joint — is not very common, lameness due to damage of the
muscular structures in the region is extremely common. Identifying the
source of this lameness requires careful examination with a Faradic
machine and treatment which not only allows repair of the injured
muscle but favours its return to full use.

Injury to the shoulder joint occurs because of direct trauma or as a
result of concussion, as in jumping. It is seen infrequently. Diagnosis

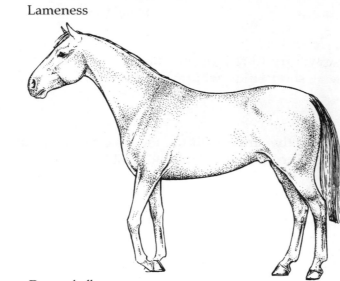

Dropped elbow

of injury to the joint is made if swelling, heat and pain can be located in the area.

Treatment will involve rest, the possible use of anti-inflammatory agents and physiotherapy to the inflamed joint.

The term 'jarred shoulders' normally describes a muscular condition as the joint itself is usually found to be healthy.

Elbow Lameness

The elbow joint is made up of the lower end of the humerus and the upper ends of the radius and ulna.

Many of the factors of shoulder lameness apply to elbow lameness — joint lameness is not common although it does occur. On occasion there is separation of the radius and ulna at the back of the elbow, and extended rest is required to resolve it.

Dropped Elbow

This condition is the result of injury to the radial nerve in the region of the shoulder. It usually occurs from a direct blow, perhaps in a fall, or by running into a hard object like a wall or fence.

Symptoms: There is dropping of the structures of the shoulder and elbow and the leg is held in a flexed position, the animal generally being unable to bring it forward. No weight is borne on the affected leg.

Diagnosis: Paralysis is reflected in restricted movement of the leg and there may be no feeling below the area of the initial injury.

Treatment: Physiotherapy aims to heal the damaged tissues and restore function to paralysed muscles. While complete severing of the nerve would present a hopeless prognosis, many of these cases are returned to full normality with proper care. Repair of nervous tissues is slow but the eventual result, in most cases, is well worth time and patience.

Carpitis

The carpus − or knee − of the horse is a complex structure consisting of three distinct articulations: 1) the radio-carpal joint formed between the lower end of the radius and the upper row of carpal bones; 2) the intercarpal joint, formed between the two rows of carpal bones; 3) the carpo-metacarpal joint, formed between the lower row of carpal bones and the upper ends of the metacarpal bones. The equine knee corresponds to the human wrist.

Carpitis is an injury to the knee involving inflammation of the joint, tearing of the ligaments, or damage to the bones within it.

Symptoms: There is swelling of the knee with heat and pain on palpation. Lameness is generally marked.

Diagnosis: X-rays are essential in any chronic swelling of the knee to eliminate the possibility of bone fractures and chips.

Treatment: Lasers and ultrasound are commonly used to relieve the symptoms and reduce inflammation of the joint. These forms of therapy are remarkably effective in arthritic conditions, and may even help to promote the repair of small bone fragments if the leg is kept immobilised.

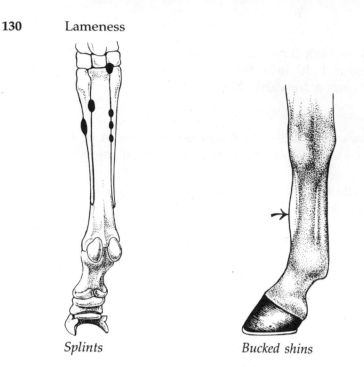

Splints   *Bucked shins*

Splints

The large metacarpal bone of the foreleg is commonly called the cannon bone. In the hind leg, the cannon is the large metatarsal bone. To either side of each large metacarpal and metatarsal, at the back, there is a smaller metacarpal or metatarsal — called the splint bone — attached to the cannon by ligament. These actually represent vestigial digits — fingers — because the cannon bone and the bones beneath it represent a single digit of the human hand or foot.

The development of bone in the horse is not complete until the horse is at least four years old, and the bonding of splint bones to the cannon takes the same time. Most splint lameness occurs in younger horses, though it can be a problem in horses of all ages.

Splints are seen as hard bony swellings found between the splint and cannon bones. They may be single or numerous, small or extensive.

Concussion is a causative factor, as are nutritional problems affecting the formation of bone, such as deficiencies of vitamins A, D and E, calcium, magnesium, and phosphorus. The balance of the leg is critical in this condition; it is important to ensure that the feet are level and that shoeing ensures a good angulation of the foot with the ground at the point of impact.

Diagnosis: Lameness from splints is aggravated on rough ground or when a horse is asked to trot downhill. The affected limb may be splayed outwards from under the body as the horse moves. Lameness can be marked even before any bony enlargement has developed, although pressure on the splint area may well expose pain at this time.

By lifting the leg, with the knee flexed, a splint may be felt between the edge of the suspensory ligament and the splint bone. If it is just developing, it may be soft and spongy. There may be heat, and the horse will respond to slight pressure with evident pain.

Many splints form without lameness. On palpation they are hard and cold.

It should be noted that many animals show varying degrees of sensitivity to handling. A distinction needs to be made between reactions to pain and objections to handling.

Treatment: With younger horses, rest will encourage the splint to harden, and it is vital to ensure that the balance of the feet is attended to.

Using anti-inflammatory drugs for this condition is unwise, the cause has to be established and rectified. If it is a nutritional problem, the animal may become sound when it is corrected, but the splint may remain for life. Where the splint is due to faulty foot care, correction may well see it regress.

Blistering and firing of splints has been done, but there is no evidence to indicate that either advances the healing process in any way. The condition responds to corrective shoeing better than to any other form of therapy.

Sore Shins

This is an inflammation of the periosteum — the outer bone covering — of the large metacarpal and metatarsal bones, although it is more common in the forelegs. In extreme cases there is swelling when the condition is described as 'bucked shin'. In all cases the shins are very tender to handle, and many affected horses pick up their legs in anticipation of pain when approached.

Usually no gross abnormality of the bone is seen, though it will have an obvious convexity in profile when the shin is bucked. The condition is common in two- and three-year-old racehorses and is due to the effect of concussion on the immature bone. It is also a problem in older horses, and some are predisposed to it throughout their racing lives. The problem is more commonly induced by hard ground, though some horses appear to suffer most on soft-to-holding surfaces. It is found in young Arab horses that work on soft ground only, and horses ridden on hard, flat beaches are prone to it.

Diagnosis: The condition is suspected where the animal is seen to shorten his stride on ground that does not suit him. When the shins are handled after work the animal will exhibit acute pain.

Treatment: While rest is effective — horses do not come in from grass suffering from this condition — the demands of training mean that fit horses are unlikely to be turned out for a condition which appears relatively insignificant. While all sorts of surface treatments are used, laser and ultrasound therapy are the most effective for relieving the symptoms. However it must be appreciated that the injury is a serious one and the periosteum is, in many cases, separated from the under-lying bone.

While these forms of treatment are effective in reducing inflammation and pain, it does not mean the underlying problem is resolved. Horses may continue to perform while under treatment but the healing process will take time to complete.

In the past, fractures of the cannon have been said to have resulted from treatment of sore shins with ultrasound; there is no scientific proof to support this. The problem may have arisen from relieving the pain while not curing the condition. Repair of bone injuries takes time, irrespective of treatment.

Many older horses eventually have to be turned out before the condition heals fully.

Sesamoiditis

In the anatomy of the fetlock joint, besides the cannon and the first pastern bones, there are two smaller bones which articulate at the back of the cannon and are known as proximal sesamoids. They act as a

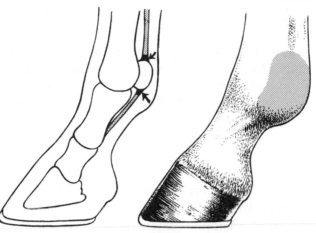

Sesamoiditis

fulcrum to the flexor tendons where these pass over their hind surface, within a synovial sheath, on the way down to the foot. The suspensory ligament is attached to the sesamoids; they are attached to each other and to the lower end of the cannon and the first pastern bone by numerous ligaments. It is a complex area and liable to injury.

Through concussion, overextension, twists and sprains, the sesamoid bones may be injured and become inflamed. The reaction to injury may lead to considerable swelling in the area and this swelling may further complicate movement. The ligaments attached to the sesamoids may be torn away, bringing with them small pieces of the bone. Because of the dependent anatomy of the region, lameness can become chronic. The ends tend to pull apart and are unable to knit. Treatment has to be aimed at counteracting this effect.

Symptoms: An animal is always lame with sesamoid injury. In the immediate aftermath, there will be heat and swelling, though this will tend to reduce with time. It may not be possible to pinpoint pain to the area if the leg is manipulated manually – and it should be stressed that overvigorous efforts to do this will only aggravate the condition. However the continued presence of heat is significant, even when all other signs of injury have abated. The area of heat is confined to the back and sides of the fetlock. The condition usually develops as the result of a strain or twist to the joint. It is typical of what might happen when a horse places his foot in a hole.

Diagnosis: This needs to be supported by x-rays.

Treatment: If lameness is acute the joint is immobilised with a tight supporting bandage. Corrective shoeing, elevating the heels, will help relieve the tension on the sesamoids. This support will need to be kept up for a period of weeks, and during that time laser or ultrasound therapy will usually effect a complete cure.

Pastern

The pastern is the area between the lower end of the fetlock and the foot. It is made up of the first and second phalanges, the latter articulating with the third phalanx (or pedal bone) and navicular bone within the hoof.

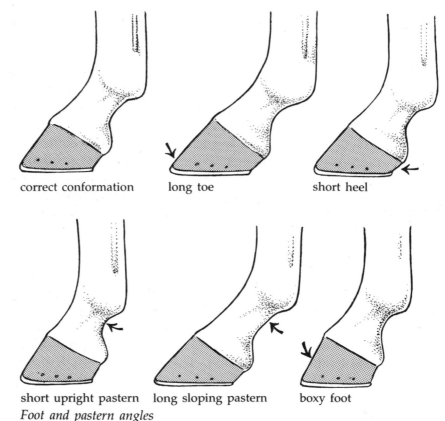

correct conformation   long toe   short heel

short upright pastern long sloping pastern   boxy foot

Foot and pastern angles

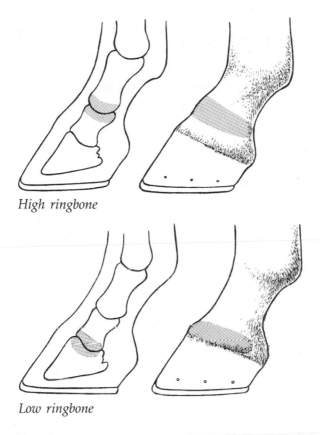

High ringbone

Low ringbone

Ringbone

While the incidence of this condition has declined in modern times — because of the different usage of horses nowadays — it is still common, usually as a result of direct trauma rather than concussion. Ringbone is described as high or low, depending on whether it occurs at the centre of the pastern or in the region of the coronet. The swelling is due to damage to the periosteum and/or a joint in the area. If it impinges on a joint or where a tendon moves over the bone, the lameness is more serious.

It is seen in either fore or hind legs in the young racehorse, and can finish the animal's racing career. While formerly it occurred as a result of concussion of the forelegs in heavy or aged horses, this picture has substantially changed now; it is seen more commonly as a sprain of the structures in the area.

Diagnosis: There is often a gross reaction with heat and swelling when the injury occurs at exercise. It is vital that any such injury be x-rayed in order to locate underlying fractures. In more chronic cases, the stride is shortened and the lameness accentuated on rough ground or when the animal is turned sharply.

Treatment: Less serious injuries may be relieved with rest, but with more serious ones which involve joints, it is difficult to return the horse to full working soundness.

Modern deep treatment with ultrasound, lasers and magnetic field therapy offers great scope for uncomplicated healing in areas of acute bony and ligamentous damage, but it is important that the problem be tackled early and pursued to a satisfactory conclusion. Inevitably the cost of doing this has to be weighed against other factors.

When the injury ends with fusion of two bones through a joint, as long as there is no pain on movement, the animal may continue to function adequately but with a somewhat altered gait.

Laminitis

To appreciate this condition you must first understand the structure of the foot. On the inner surface of the wall are about 600 leaves, or laminae, which interlock with corresponding laminae covering the front of the pedal bone. This interlocking holds the pedal bone in position more or less suspended above the frog. These leaves have a substantial blood supply and, in consequence, should anything occur to suddenly increase the flow of blood to the foot, congestion occurs. Unlike soft tissues, the hoof is unable to expand. The laminae become swollen and are forced apart, especially at the toe, but those at the heel often remain interlocked. The toe of the pedal bone, having lost its attachments, drops, presses on the sole and causes the latter to become flat or even convex. The condition can affect all four feet.

The causes are infectious and noninfectious and there is acute pain due to pressure on the sensitive laminae. It can result from concussion, although this is not typical of the condition seen today which is more often associated with feeding. Small ponies notoriously suffer when allowed free access to grass. It can result from overfeeding, from dietary changes and as a result of toxic conditions. In the mare, it may result from retention of the afterbirth.

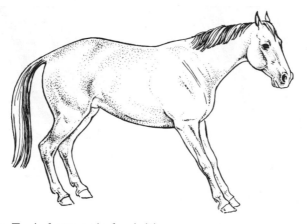

Typical stance in laminitis

Symptoms: These are divided into acute and chronic forms.

Acute — This appears suddenly and the animal is unable to move without great pain. If only the forelegs are affected the animal gets his hind feet in under his body to relieve the weight on the forelegs. This stance may confuse an owner into thinking the animal is suffering from a problem in the back. If the horse is made to turn, it will appear that the forelegs are being lifted off the ground after which the feet are placed down gently at the heels.

There may be sweating and a rise in temperature. Heat will be felt in affected feet.

Chronic — Chronic cases are often the aftereffect of acute attacks. The level of pain is less, but heat is still detectable in the foot and the animal suffers at all gaits. He bears weight on his heel and there is a gradual change in the shape of the foot. The toe elongates and turns upwards and the heel and pastern respond accordingly. The sole flattens and the tip of the pedal bone may press down on it, occasionally penetrating through.

Treatment: Veterinary advice is necessary in all acute cases. The cause of the problem needs to be identified and removed.

Early efforts are made to reduce pain and relieve the symptoms. The animal may be placed in a stream to foster this. Alternatively cold hosing or applying ice-packs may help.

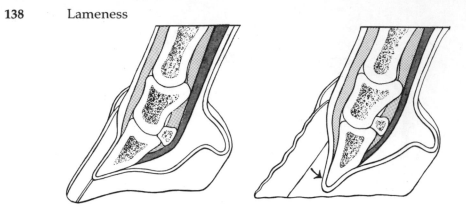

Rotation of pedal bone in laminitis: normal foot (left), rotation of pedal bone (right)

When small ponies are affected it is necessary to remove them from the source of their problem – grass. Careful attention to their feet must be given by an experienced farrier.

Laminitis in Thoroughbreds is normally satisfactorily reversed by relieving the symptoms and removing the cause. The use of a good purgative is a significant help.

In chronic cases, care of the feet is paramount, and it is necessary, by even rigorous trimming, to restore normal shape to feet which have become distorted. This may be done in conjunction with x-rays, to check on the rotation of the pedal bone. Corrective shoeing may help an animal to get about without pain.

Navicular Disease

In the foot, behind the pedal bone, there is a small shuttle-shaped bone called the navicular. It acts as a fulcrum for the deep flexor tendon before this is attached to the undersurface of the pedal bone – to the wings of which it is itself attached by ligaments. The navicular bone may become diseased, and the condition can later involve the deep tendon and the bursa that rests between tendon and bone. As this progresses, adhesions can form between tendon and bone, and the bone is demineralised gradually.

The causes of the condition are a combination of conformation and concussion arising from work. Contributory causes are poor frog pressure due to bad shoeing – as in contracted heels – and long toe growth allowing undue strain on the flexor tendons. It may also occur

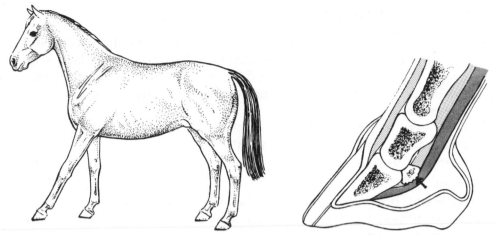

Resting stance in navicular disease; 'pointing' the foot (left). Pitting of the navicular bone (right)

as an upward extension of chronic foot infection.

Diagnosis: The condition has to be considered in all cases of foot lameness. However final confirmation is dependent on satisfactory x-ray pictures.

Navicular disease may be suspected where there is a history of intermittent lameness related to the foot. Often both feet are affected and the stride is short and choppy. At rest, affected feet may be pointed to relieve tension on the painful part. Initial lameness improves as the animal warms up. After rest the symptoms become more pronounced. The shoes of affected feet are worn at the toe.

Navicular disease is easily confused with other conditions of the lower leg. It is also worth noting that gait changes are very often associated with muscular injuries of the shoulder region.

Treatment: Numerous modern efforts have been made to treat this condition. Warfarin and isoxsuprine are used with some success.

Navicular disease has become the fashionable lameness of our times and many problems are attributed to it incorrectly.

The most rational approach to bone and ligamentous injuries of the foot is with direct forms of deep treatment, using laser or ultrasound. Pain is relieved and animals are kept in work.

Corrective shoeing aims to raise the heels and roll the toe. Pads may be fitted under the shoe to reduce concussion.

Pedal Ostitis

This is an inflammatory condition of the third phalanx caused by jarring on hard ground, leading to demineralisation. It may be a sequel to corns, laminitis or punctures of the sole. It is also more common with age, as the feet lose shape and texture, thus increasing concussion on the bone.

By its very nature pedal ostitis is slow to develop and changes may be evident on x-ray before the animal is found to be lame. There may be pain on pressure of the sole and the condition commonly affects both forefeet.

Diagnosis: This is made by x-ray. Lameness may not be marked early in the condition but increases with time and the animal moves more freely on soft surfaces.

Treatment: As the underlying condition involves demineralisation of bone, this is a difficult process to reverse. In many cases, anatomical changes which have already occurred in the foot, increasing concussion, are permanent. However, daily treatment with ultrasound or laser therapy can adequately relieve the symptoms so that the animal can be kept in work. On x-ray, this treatment can be shown to improve the condition of the bone.

Sidebones

This name describes a condition where the cartilages at either side of the foot become hard and ossified. The normal function of these cartilages, which attach to the wings of the pedal bone, is as part of the

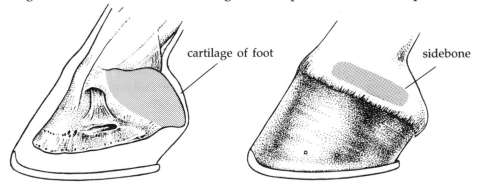

cartilage of foot

sidebone

Collateral cartilages and the position of sidebone

shock-absorbing system of the foot. When they become bony, through the effects of concussion, this facility is lost.

The condition is most common in heavy and plain-bred horses.

Diagnosis: Lameness is not a common feature of the condition. The hardened cartilages are felt at the junction of hair and hoof in the region of the quarter of the foot.

Treatment: As lameness is negligible or absent the condition is not normally treated.

Contracted Heels

The heels contract due to lack of frog pressure. This happens either because of faulty shoeing or when the wall at the heel is allowed to grow too long. It can also happen with any chronic lameness in which

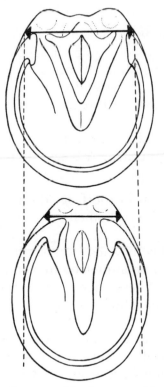

Contracted heels: normal heel (top), contracted heel (bottom)

the heel is not brought into contact with the ground. Contraction is easily seen by the naked eye and may precede overall contraction of the foot. It may happen in any foot, though more commonly in front feet. When established the problem may take some time to correct.

Diagnosis: On examination of the foot, the frog will be high and have a shrunken appearance. Where only one foot is affected, its size in comparison to its neighbour is notably smaller. The hoof will have a boxy and upright appearance. There may be drying of the wall due to the contraction of the coronary band.

Treatment: The aim is to restore frog pressure. The heels are paired down to bring them into contact with the ground. A special shoe may be designed with a pad or bar to ensure frog pressure.

Thrush

This is a degenerative condition of the frog caused by dirty wet conditions. It normally reflects poor standards of stable management, with the animal standing in rank and fetid bedding. It may occur in either fore or hind feet. The cleft of the frog is moist and evil smelling.

It is not unusual for the problem to extend through to the sensitive foot and set up infection within.

The frog itself may be undermined and the lateral grooves between frog and horn found to be deeper than normal. A black discharge may be present.

Diagnosis: This is based on the condition of the frog, the presence of excessive moisture, undermining, and the evil smell.

Treatment: The cleft of the frog should be opened back so that affected areas are exposed to air. The foot should be immersed in a solution of 5 per cent copper sulphate or formalin. Where there is infection of the sensitive foot, drainage should be established where possible. Antibiotics are indicated in severe cases.

As the condition results from poor stable hygiene, this problem is prevented by careful attention to foot health. Feet should be picked out regularly and dressed with a suitable hoof dressing. Underfoot conditions need to be dry and clean.

Canker

This is a degenerative condition of the foot caused by standing in dirty stables. It is not common today. It is marked by a soft underrun (i.e. the horn separates from the underlying structures) sole and frog. In advanced cases areas of sensitive sole may be exposed.

Symptoms: No lameness may be present in the early stages. A heavy, evil-smelling discharge comes from infected tissues.

Diagnosis: This is based on examination of the foot and exposure of the dead and rotting tissues.

Treatment: All diseased areas are pared away and infection limited by use of antiseptic and antibiotic packs. The sensitive areas must be protected until healing occurs, and this can take months to achieve.

Corns

A corn is a bruise of the sensitive foot at the angle between the wall and bar, at the heel. It is more common in forefeet where it may occur at either angle. The normal cause is the shoe bearing directly on the sole at the site of corn. Alternatively, a stone may wedge under the shoe, causing the same problem. In early corn development, the bruising may be seen and blood may be evident beneath the surface. Later, if not treated, it takes on a yellowish appearance as the tissues degenerate. Horses differ in their tendency to corns, some being prone to them. A great deal depends on the shape of the foot and texture of the horn.

Symptoms: Varying degrees of lameness, depending on the hardness of the ground. There may be heat in the region of the heels and the blood vessels on the affected side of the leg may be enlarged and pulsing. The animal tries to avoid bearing weight on the affected part. Where the corn leads to infection of the sensitive foot, lameness will be more marked.

Diagnosis: The shoe will need to be removed to expose the corn. The animal will flinch on application of pressure to the part. The damaged tissue can be seen quite clearly at the site of corn.

Treatment: The damaged tissue is pared back and, if infection has gone to the sensitive foot, drainage established. Poultices are applied to draw it off. Antibiotics may be needed in obstinate cases.

A seated-out shoe should be fitted to avoid further pressure on the site. Care needs to be taken with future shoeing as the condition may recur. In some cases a threequarter shoe will be necessary to allow the damaged tissue to grow back.

Prevention of tetanus is wise in any case of infection of the foot.

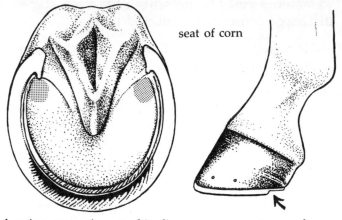

seat of corn

seedy toe showing separation at white line   cutaway shoe

Seat of corn and cutaway shoe

Seedy Toe

In this condition the wall of the foot separates from the sole at the white line. The space formed is filled with a soft crumbling horn. It is often associated with chronic laminitis. Infection may enter through this path. The condition becomes evident at shoeing and does not produce lameness.

The dead horn is trimmed out and prevention of infection is promoted by packing with tow impregnated with a mild antiseptic or sulphanilamide powder. Attention should also be given to the diet to ensure proper horn growth.

Sandcrack

This condition involves cracks in the wall of the hoof running between the ground and coronet. These may be partial or complete, penetrating

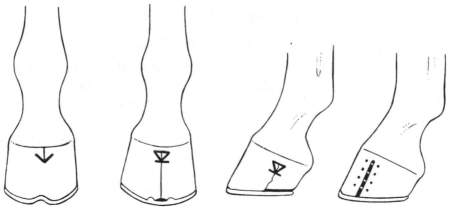

Sandcrack: position of cracks on feet and treatment

through the full thickness of the wall at times. They are caused by injury, or defects in growth at the coronary band. Lameness is evident in serious cases. Sandcracks may occur in any foot and are seen at the toe, quarter or heel.

Symptoms: Horses coming in from grass will invariably have cracks if the ground is dry and hard and the feet have not been regularly trimmed. These will travel part way up the wall and cause little trouble when the horse is shod. However if the crack opens on contact with the ground, lameness is likely to occur.

Diagnosis: It is important to determine the cause and extent of the crack. If it is due to damage to the coronary band, treatment will have to be aimed at this area.

Treatment: Where the crack does not extend the whole length of the wall, a groove or pattern burned into the top will immobilise it and facilitate healing. A shoe clip may be used for the same purpose. Should the crack reach the end of the wall it must be trimmed back so that the break does not come in contact with the shoe or ground.

Some deep cracks are filled with plastics to prevent the sensitive tissues from being damaged.

Where it is necessary to promote horn growth, the hoof is dressed daily in hoof oil, and mineral mixes are given which provide the essential nutrients needed.

Coronary band injuries respond well to ultrasound and laser therapy.

Hind Leg Lameness

Stifle Slip (Upward Fixation of the Patella)

The stifle joint is composed of the lower end of the femur, the upper end of the tibia, and the patella. It correlates with the knee joint of man and actually consists of two joints — the femoro-patellar joint, between the femur and the patella, and the femoro-tibial joint, between the femur and tibia. This latter joint includes two cartilages, known as articular menisci, or semilunar cartilages.

The condition is marked by dislocation of the patella, the bone that corresponds to the human knee cap. The patella is seated naturally in a groove at the end of the femur and is held in position by a number of ligaments. In upward fixation it slips out of the groove onto the medial condyle of the bone. This is often thought to have an hereditary predisposition, but it occurs in a number of different circumstances. It is more likely in legs with an upright angulation of the stifle. Poor condition also seems to predispose to it.

Once it has occurred, the stretching of the ligaments makes it more likely to happen again. It may occur in only one hind leg, but it is possible for both limbs to be affected.

Symptoms: The leg is locked in extension and the horse will generally refuse to bear weight on the affected limb. The stifle and hock cannot flex, but the fetlock can. The locking may last for hours or only moments. In some cases it keeps happening and relieving itself. If the horse is forced to move it will drag the affected foot along the ground. A typical clicking sound may be heard when the patella is released.

Diagnosis: The symptom of rigid extension of a hind leg is typical, and the problem is not relieved until the animal manages to free the fixed patella — possibly by a sudden movement. The condition can occur in animals of all ages from yearling upwards.

Treatment: By putting a sideline on the affected limb and lifting it forward towards the neck the patella may be released. Direct pressure on the patella itself may help return it to its natural position. The bedding should subsequently be of paper or shavings to help the animal get around the stable with ease.

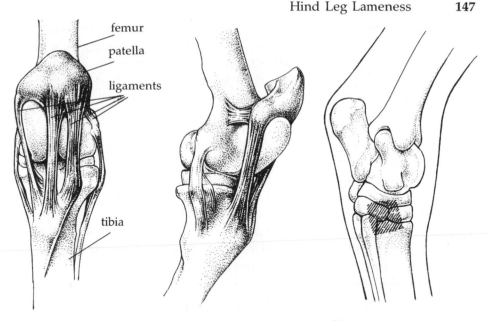

Stifle: front view   *Stifle: side view*   *Site of spavin*

Anti-inflammatory drugs will help keep the reaction within the stifle to a minimum.

Surgery is performed on older horses with a recurrent history of this problem. The results of the operation are good.

Spavin

The hock joint is a complex structure consisting of the six small tarsal bones and their articulation with the tibia above, with each other, and with the large metatarsal bone below. There are, therefore, three articulations involved, namely, the tibio-tarsal, the intertarsal, and the tarso-metatarsal.

Spavin is the cause of bony enlargement on the inner side of the hock due to inflammation in the area. It can involve the upper end of the cannon bone and the bones and joints of the hock nearby. The result may be arthritis and fusion of the affected bones.

The condition is related to poor hock conformation, perhaps coupled with concussive injury to the area. When formed, bone spavin is readily recognised at the junction of the lower end of the hock and the beginning of the cannon bone on the inner side of the leg.

Symptoms: Lameness is most pronounced when trotting from standing; it diminishes with exercise. In the early stages, the animal may become lame following a period of rest after fast work. The action of the affected limb may be altered, with wear on the outside of the shoe. Flexion of the joint may be reduced and the horse will track short on the affected side.

Diagnosis: Spavin is confirmed on finding the typical swelling on the inside of the hock. Even in early cases where the bone has not increased in size, heat will be marked over the site of spavin.

Picking the leg up and flexing it for anything longer than thirty seconds is the basis of the 'spavin test'. When the limb is released the horse is trotted away and lameness is marked if the horse has spavin. However, this test is not specific and other sources of lameness will be accentuated through the same process.

The condition is confirmed by x-ray.

Treatment: Spavin does not respond well to treatment and tends to be progressive once developed. Rest and other treatments may well alleviate the signs but if the horse is returned to full work the condition usually recurs. It is not uncommon for both legs to be affected, even sequentially.

Surgery for the condition is quite effective. Corrective shoeing is aimed at balancing the foot when it lands on the ground.

In many cases the horse remains technically unsound but is able to continue work.

Occult (or Blind) Spavin is the name for spavin lameness with no bony swelling.
Jack Spavin is a large bone spavin.
High Spavin is located higher on the hock than normal bone spavin.
Bog Spavin is a chronic swelling of the hock joint with soft swelling on the front and back of the hock.

Slipping of the Superficial Flexor Tendon off the Hock

This condition is mostly seen in racehorses. It may be linked with poor conformation and occurs most commonly during the course of a jumping race.

Symptoms: There is marked lameness and swelling of the point of the hock.

Diagnosis: The early signs may not easily be distinguished from capped hock, though, as the swelling reduces, the abnormal placing of the superficial flexor tendon — which can occur to either side — is seen. It must not be confused with rupture of the Achilles tendon at the point of the hock or damage to other structures of the joint.

Treatment: Surgery is necessary if the animal is to return to working soundness.

Stringhalt

This is marked by an abnormal spasmodic action of the hind leg when lifted from the ground. It may be seen when the animal is walking or when moving over in the stable. It can affect one or both hind legs and is usually constant once it has appeared, though intermittent types are described. Although the cause is unknown, it is thought to have a nervous origin.

Symptoms: The leg tends to shake involuntarily when flexed. In some cases the first steps are exaggerated before the animal finds his stride. The symptoms are more marked when turning short or backing.

Diagnosis: The action of the leg is typical and cannot be easily confused with any other condition. However varying degrees of abnormality are seen and in the early stages may be only slight. It must not be confused with upward fixation of the patella, where there is rigid extension of the limb while the patella is trapped, or with muscular injuries which affect action.

Treatment: Surgery is performed though its success is limited. The condition is progressive but many horses manage to continue a useful ridden existence and even race with stringhalt.

Shivering

This condition is marked by abnormal movements of the hind legs and tail. Occasionally the forelegs are affected. The symptoms suggest a nervous origin.

Symptoms: When horses are only slightly affected, nothing may be noted when they are standing still or moving forward. A false movement may be detected when the horse moves over in his stable or when he is asked to turn short or back. The tail may rise and quiver, a leg may be raised off the ground and held up. The horse may tend to lose balance, and when asked to back, may be unable to do so properly.

Diagnosis: This is often very difficult in early stages but the typical movement of the tail and hind legs, especially when the animal is asked to back, is peculiar to the condition. More advanced cases merge with symptoms of conditions such as *wobbling*, in which there are often lesions of the spinal cord.

Treatment: There is no treatment and the condition is progressive.

Sprains of Tendons and Ligaments

Because of the dynamic nature of the horse and the special limitations of his leg anatomy, injury to tendons and ligaments has a particular importance. Injury is common to all kinds of ridden horses − though mostly to the racehorse.

Tendons differ from ligaments in texture and function, but their place in the anatomy and physiology of the leg has much common ground.

Tendons

A tendon is not a separate entity, but an extension of the fleshy part of a muscle. It is strong and fibrous, and is attached to bone at its distal end. The fleshy part of the muscle is elastic and capable of contraction and relaxation. The tendon has little elasticity and is almost rigid when compared with the muscle.

Muscle fibre is more delicate and more capable of being strained. The difference in their respective healing properties, however, makes injury to a tendon a great deal more serious.

The most common site of injury is on the flexors of the foreleg, in the area between the back of the knee and the fetlock. Different structures may be damaged here and the degree of injury varies from mild bruising to complete rupture of tendon fibres.

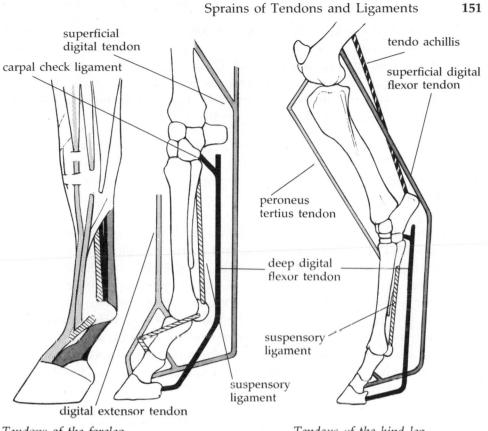

Tendons of the foreleg

Tendons of the hind leg

Causes:

    a. Overuse when the horse is unfit. This includes the common mistake of trying to get horses fit too quickly.

    b. False ground (i.e. ground that varies from firm to soft).

    c. Hard ground.

    d. Jumping drop fences.

    e. Slipping up.

    f. Bad conformation — long weak pasterns, back at the knee, poorly-made tendons.

    g. Muscular injury, as this reduces the elasticity of the muscle/tendon unit and alters the shape of the leg.

    h. Overreaches.

It is likely that tendons are far more durable than we give them credit for. They are much more likely to be damaged, however, when a horse is not fit enough for the task in hand. Under normal circumstances it is the fleshy part of the muscle that absorbs any shock or strain the leg is subjected to. When a muscle is damaged, the muscle/tendon relationship is altered, so increasing strain on the tendon.

Symptoms: Is is advised to study the accompanying sketches carefully, and to learn the different anatomical structures of the area involved. Then, by reference to the leg of a living horse, define the individual tendons, even picking the leg from the ground and feeling the divisions between them.

A slight strain may affect the sheath and fibres of the superficial flexor tendon only, resulting in heat and a little swelling. There may be no lameness, but if the leg is picked up and the area subjected to slight finger pressure, pain will be noted. It is important to distinguish between real pain and the resentment some horses show to any applied pressure. Where there is an injury the pain will be confined to the area in which there is heat. If in doubt, compare the reaction in a sound leg.

A more severe strain with rupture of fibres will cause greater swelling, which may give the leg a bowed appearance and span most of the length of the tendon. Lameness is often present at the walk and pain is marked on finger pressure.

Rupture of a whole tendon will cause the fetlock to be dropped below its normal position.

If both the superficial and deep tendons are ruptured, the fetlock will have lost the greater part of its support and may drop almost to the level of the ground. The horse will be in acute distress and the pain will cause it to sweat and blow.

Diagnosis: The presence of heat in a tendon is a warning at any time that there is a weakness. Trainers feel the tendons and joints of their horses every evening to detect early signs of injury and horses found to have any heat are given special care. The more advanced injuries cannot easily be mistaken.

It is common today to examine injured tendons with diagnostic ultrasonic scanners.

Treatment: There is a great deal of controversy over the treatment of

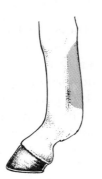

Common area of tendon damage

tendon injuries, especially when the condition is chronic. Recent moves by the Royal College of Veterinary Surgeons to ban the firing of horses have been criticised as well as welcomed.

With any tendon injury it has to be appreciated that the mechanics of leg anatomy tends to draw the injured ends apart. For this reason support of the injury by firm bandaging is vital. Efforts to limit the inflammation are widely varied. While some use hot poultices others use ice and cold-hosing. Some use anti-inflammatory drugs, which may be necessary to control reaction and pain in severe cases.

Whichever method used, the initial inflammatory response has to be controlled. Bandaging will help to limit swelling; in many cases this support is withdrawn too early and the problem is made worse.

Allowing nature to take its course is not a wise move with this condition.

The greatest problem with slight tendon injuries arises when horses are returned to work too soon, before the leg has had time to repair. There are occasions when animals with serious tendon injuries continue to race effectively – however they are so few as to be a distortion of reality. Every injury to this area should be taken seriously and each step of the return to work watched carefully.

When a leg is being bandaged, ensure pressure is applied evenly and, in addition, the fetlock must be supported when the injury is near the joint. Cotton wool or gauze should be used under nonadhesive support bandages to prevent interference with blood supply. When using adhesive bandages it is vital to avoid wrinkling or twisting of the bandage material. It is also wise to give support to both injured and sound legs in order to avoid damage to the weight-bearing leg.

A wedge-heel shoe may be applied for the first few weeks to relieve tension on the tendon.

After about two to three days, the injured area can be treated with ultrasound or laser therapies. However it is important to keep the initial treatment levels low and to only treat the perimeters of the injury because pain can be provoked by treatment at this stage. As time progresses, the level can be increased and the treatment head brought directly over the injury. This is by far the most effective way of getting a good repair with minimal swelling.

When the heat has gone and the animal is sound he should be turned out and given a period of not less than six months rest before being returned to work. This is because the healing of tendon tissue takes considerable time to complete.

As aforementioned, tendon injuries are very often preceded by muscular damage. It is critical if this has happened that the muscle be treated before the horse is put back in work, otherwise the condition is almost certain to recur.

It can be stated with authority that the best results with injured tendons are achieved through intelligent use of modern physiotherapeutic means. The cause of the initial injury has to be established and, where possible, avoided, but the majority of horses will continue to race sound if the mechanics of the condition, and the animal, are fully taken into account.

While a variety of mild blisters may be used when the horse is out, their effect is largely palliative. Control of the initial reaction will prevent adhesions and excessive swellings. Time will restore the tendon to its former strength. The return to work must be slow and patient, with plenty of basic slow-pace exercise before the animal canters.

There can be no case in favour of firing tendons as the results from well-managed physiotherapy are better. Most surgical and injection techniques fail because of a lack of understanding of the cause, furthermore, any procedure which leaves the animal with a visible swelling on the tendon is unlikely to provide the strength to withstand training.

Ligaments

A ligament differs from a tendon in not having a muscular body attached to it. It is also less elastic and its function is to hold bones together or act as a support to a joint.

The suspensory ligament — This is attached to the back of the cannon bone in the groove formed between this bone and the splint bones to either side. Just above the sesamoids it sends two branches forward to joint the extensor tendons on the front of the pastern. The rest of the ligament is attached to the sesamoids. Its function is to suspend the fetlock and support the leg. The suspensory ligament is a part of the stay apparatus.

Injury to the suspensory ligament occurs as a primary injury, probably due to overextension of the fetlock joint. Hard ground is also a cause of injury to this ligament.

Symptoms: There is diffuse swelling of the full tendon area and pain on palpation of the suspensory. The horse will be lame and have a short choppy stride at the trot.

Diagnosis: Heat and swelling are marked on the ligament, which will be felt more easily with the leg picked up. There is no bowing of the outer tendons and no pain when the flexors are subjected to finger pressure. Pain is marked when the suspensory itself is handled. It usually has a soft feeling to it when compared with the ligament of a sound leg.

It is important not to confuse tendon and ligament injuries with infection of the same area, which can be equally painful.

Treatment: Support by bandaging is important initially together with other measures to limit pain and control the extent of the inflammatory process. After the first two days the ligament may be treated with deep physiotherapy and the horse will usually return to work within six weeks.

The carpal check ligament — This is a short ligament that extends from the back of the knee — or carpus — to the deep flexor tendon, halfway down the cannon bone. It supports the deep tendon and also plays a part in the stay apparatus which helps to keep an animal in a standing position while resting. There is also a *radial check ligament* which is part of the same apparatus, however it is less commonly involved in lameness.

The most likely cause of injury is sudden overextension of the knee.

Symptoms: Lameness is not very marked, the horse tending to prop slightly and shorten his stride on the affected leg.

Diagnosis: Heat is detected at the back of the knee and there is pain on manipulation of the injured ligament.

Treatment: The condition responds well to either ultrasound or laser therapy. The horse should not be ridden until all heat has gone from the area because the structures at the back of the knee are under constant strain. It is difficult to support this ligament, so rest and judicious exercise are important.

Curb

This is a strain of the ligament binding the hock to the cannon bone at the back of the leg. It is defined as any deviation in a straight line from the point of the hock to the fetlock, situated at the lower end of the hock. Strain of the ligament is frequently followed by bony enlargement. The swelling is best seen with the leg viewed from the side.

If the head of the splint bone is enlarged or positioned slightly behind the perpendicular line, this does not constitute a curb.

Badly made hocks are predisposed to the condition which occurs as a result of overextension of the joint.

Symptoms: Lameness may be noted in the early stages but it is short-lived and mild in character. The condition occurs mostly in younger horses which are not well developed or are unfit for the task in hand. It may occur as a result of immature animals being jumped too soon.

Diagnosis: The typical swelling will be found on the midline at the lower end of the back of the hock. There will be heat and pain initially but this soon passes. The enlargement may become bony and continue to grow if the hock is weak and under continued strain.

Treatment: Many curbs require no treatment, although the swelling involved is considered to be a serious blemish for showing purposes and owners will request treatment for this reason. Early swelling is best treated with ultrasound or laser, and the hock should not be subjected

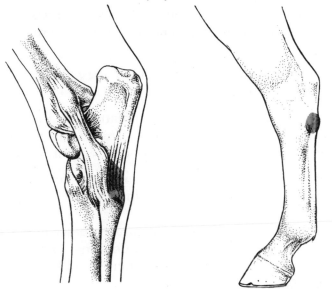

Site of ligament sprain in curb (left), point of curb (right)

to any sudden strains until all heat has gone from the site. Larger swellings with poorly made hocks and bony invasion of the curb are unlikely to be improved by any form of treatment. As long as the animal is riding sound the problem is best ignored.

Injury to Bursae, Sheaths and Joints

Bursae and sheaths are anatomical structures designed to reduce friction. They possess synovial-type lining membranes which secrete a fluid — similar in nature to joint fluid. Where a tendon, ligament or muscle passes over a bone, bursae are interposed as buffers to prevent damage to either structure. Injury usually occurs as a result of direct pressure, perhaps following injury to neighbouring parts with a consequent change of action. This is marked by swelling of the bursa and pain on manipulation.

Capped hock — This is an enlargement of the bursa at the point of the hock, and may result from banging the hock against a wall or partition.

Capped elbow — Occurs at the point of the elbow.

Bursitis may occur in a host of other situations and is particularly common on the back, where ligament or muscle overlies bony prominences.

Sheaths are found around tendons, which they protect from wear and friction by their fluid secretion.

Thoroughpin — Thoroughpin is an inflammation of the deep flexor tendon sheath near the point of the hock. This is not to be confused with bog spavin which involves the lining of the joint itself.

Windgalls — These are found in the region of the fetlocks — usually above and behind — and may involve tendon-sheaths, bursae or joints.

Symptoms: Swelling of the affected structure with accompanying pain and lameness in acute cases. However conditions such as windgalls and thoroughpin commonly settle down. There is no lameness, though the swellings remain.

These may occur when young animals are overused, in which case they are a warning to exercise caution. In mature animals they are seen as blemishes only and have little clinical significance.

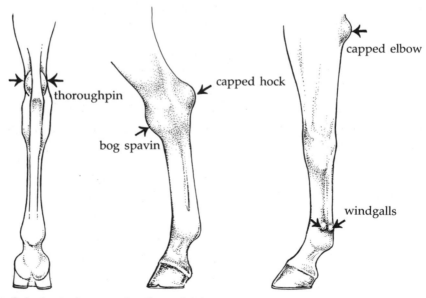

Injuries to bursae, sheaths and joints

Diagnosis: Soft swellings with pain over bony prominences tend to limit use of an animal and are of special concern in the saddle area. Fluid in a joint will hamper movement early on, though many animals are found to be functionally sound with settled enlarged joints.

Treatment: These swellings are effectively treated, when fresh, with laser and ultrasound; they reduce quickly and remain healed. Windgalls on older horses may not respond and are best left untreated when there is no lameness present.

Permanent swellings which interfere with movement are best treated, even if the animal is not continually lame. In cases involving the hock or knee, the fluid may need to be drawn off and the joint injected with an anti-inflammatory drug.

Where infection enters any of these structures — either as a result of direct trauma, or in fistulous withers (where the infecting organisms may arrive through the blood) antibiotic treatment must kill infection before other measures are taken. Instruments such as laser and ultrasound are potentially dangerous in the presence of infection.

Muscular Injuries

These are common on the neck, shoulders, back, quarters and thighs; they are less common on the gaskin and forearm.

The larger muscle bodies are more often torn, and this occurs in the early stages of training before the animal is fully fit. It results from asking the muscle to bear too great a load before it is physically ready. Tearing can also occur due to sudden unbalanced movement, or through direct trauma such as a kick.

A great deal of muscular injuries go undiagnosed and untreated. This leads to secondary lameness of tendons and joints, because the action is changed as a result of the muscle injury. The long-term effect is wasting of damaged muscle and often a chronic history of secondary lameness.

Symptoms: The horse is lame immediately after tearing a muscle but this passes off within days as other muscles in the limb compensate and take over its functions.

Diagnosis: There is swelling of the injured area but this is best detected with the use of a Faradic machine, which is both diagnostic and therapeutic. Muscular injuries seldom self-cure and the animal will have a permanently altered action if the condition is not treated.

Lameness after the initial injury, when the animal nods on contact with the ground, is not marked. However, there is lameness in movement, the action of the limb being inhibited at the trot. This is known as 'swinging-leg lameness' − as opposed to 'supporting-leg lameness'. With the latter, pain is related to concussion.

Treatment: Faradic therapy, perhaps combined with laser or ultrasound treatment to help relieve damaged tissue. Faradic stimulation is essential to restoring muscle to full use.

Back Lameness

There is wide recognition of the part played by back lameness in horses, especially those which compete and jump. The problem is often due to pressure on nerves as a result of minor movements in the spinal support structures.

Symptoms: These vary with the part of the spine involved and the nerves affected. Lameness may be marked or the action of the horse may only be marginally altered. It is not unusual for two legs on one diagonal to be unsound.

Diagnosis: The action is similar to muscular lameness, with shortening of the stride of affected limbs. The horse may not be nodding when the limb strikes the ground though movement is perceptibly altered. Diagnosis and location of the lesion is based on manipulation of the spinal column.

Treatment: Manipulation effectively restores full movement to affected limbs. Any muscular injury related to the problem is treated as before. Some animals are predisposed to this kind of lameness and are manipulated routinely as a preventive. Many good horses have back problems which seriously affect their performance, but they are controlled by constant vigilance and care.

Fractures

Fractures have to be suspected in all acute injuries where there is great pain and the animal is not inclined to put weight on the affected limb. Where there is a clean break in a large bone the diagnosis is easily made, but partial fractures of even the cannon bone without separation will require x-rays to confirm an opinion.

Treatment: Repair of large bones is limited by the nature of the animal and the difficulties imposed by the mechanics of bone fracture. Temperamentally, horses are not disposed to being held in slings while their bones mend, and the physical limitations of bone repair mean the part must be immobilised if there is to be success.

Horses are put down to save them from pain and the anxiety and shock they suffer with broken bones. This is done when the exact nature of the injury is known and a decision is made that it would be more cruel to keep the animal alive. There is no justification for subjecting an animal to continued suffering if the end result is not going to allow it a fully useful life.

Fractures of small bones like those of the pasterns, sesamoids, knee and hock, are regularly repaired successfully, and animals returned to full work. Even bad pelvic fractures with crepitating sounds audible on movement will repair if the animal is confined and rested. Other long-bone fractures are also occasionally repaired through surgery.

It is important in all cases that professional opinion be sought, allowing a proper decision to be made when the facts are assessed.

18   Care of Feet and Shoeing

That constant care of feet is vital is recognised in the old adage 'No foot, no horse'. This applies equally to the foal and yearling as to any animal out at grass. The balancing of feet in younger horses can decide the kind of legs they will have for the remainder of their lives. Unshod feet in older horses are often brittle and tend to break on dry ground.

The art of shoeing is to make the shoe fit the foot. Where this is not done there is a constant risk of ensuing lameness.

When horses are turned out to grass they are very often left without shoes. Some may have light front shoes, though there are occasions when owners will decide the feet need a complete rest from trimming and nailing. In all cases it is important to trim regularly to avoid problems when the horse comes back in. Hind shoes are best left off to avoid serious injury from kicking. Foot care should be undertaken on a monthly basis.

Points to Note

a. The feet of foals and yearlings should be trimmed regularly. This is done in conjunction with the observation of foot and leg balance. Corrections are made where the wear is uneven or the animal is developing an abnormal gait.

b. Always check for loose shoes when cleaning the feet of ridden horses. Watch for raised clenches or missing nails.

c. Ensure that the shoe has not moved and is not bearing on the sensitive sole.

d. Make sure the branches are not pressing on the site of corn.

e. Watch for hoof texture and cracks. Dress with hoof oil on a daily basis. Feed nutritional supplements where there are known deficiencies and where horn growth is faulty.

f. Horses that go lame after shoeing may have been pricked by

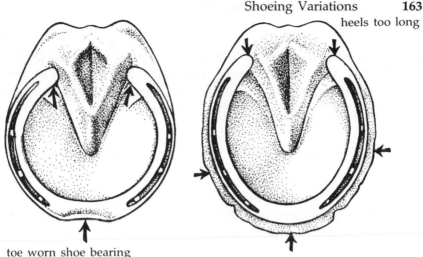

heels too long

toe worn shoe bearing
on the sole

wall of foot beyond shoe

Foot and shoeing problems

a nail inside the white line. Take precautions against foot infection and tetanus. It may be necessary to remove the shoe and poultice until soundness returns. However, where the shoe is simply tight, this may pass off — lameness will be less marked on soft surfaces.

g. Where an animal is brushing, the shoe can be receded at the point of contact, and the part being struck protected with a boot or bandage.

h. It is important to understand the anatomy of the foot and the basic dynamics of action. In this way you can appreciate problems with shoeing and help your farrier to correct them.

i. Watch for signs of thrush development or contraction of the frog.

j. Have shoes removed monthly and worn shoes replaced as the farrier advises.

Shoeing Variations

The normal shoe for riding horses is an iron shoe, oval in shape with flat bearing surface, fullered, and consisting of two branches — divided into heel and quarter — and a toe. Racing plates may be made of light iron or aluminium.

Tips

These are half shoes made of light iron which cover the toe and quarter only. They are used for protecting the horn of horses at grass, or for giving height to the toe when it is required to lower the heels. In the latter case the tip is wedge-shaped from front to rear.

Threequarter Shoes

One branch is shortened in order to avoid pressure on an injured part. Alternatively, they are often used for yearlings and foals to correct a developing imbalance of the foot. For this purpose either branch may be missing and the shoe is lowered gradually from one end to the other.

Feather-edged Shoes

These are used to prevent brushing. The inner branch of the fore or hind shoe is narrowed to avoid striking the opposite limb.

Wedge-heeled Shoes

The heel is raised to relieve pressure on injured tendons, joints or ligaments. It is important to remember that the recovered limb will need time to adjust when the shoe is removed.

Leather Padding

This is used to reduce concussion and protect the sole or frog from bruising.

Wedge-shaped Plastic Pads

These are used for sole protection and to give height to the heels where needed. They are often used for horses with long sloping pasterns to effectively reduce the angle of the foot with the ground.

The pads need to be removed regularly as dirt and stones may get underneath them.

Anti-slipping Devices

Studs are probably the most efficient way of preventing slipping. They are the choice in countries where horses travel on ice and snow. They are normally combined with toe-grabs to retain the proper foot axis with the ground.

Some shoes are made with an anti-slip bearing surface, but, a problem in some cases is that the shoes wear unevenly and the horse is left on a shoe that rocks, leading to possible joint trouble.

Plastic Shoes

These are fitted when there is a problem with normal shoeing — perhaps due to bruising, or inadequate room for nails. The plastic shoes are bonded to the feet and give good wear for about a month. They are a solution to many foot problems.

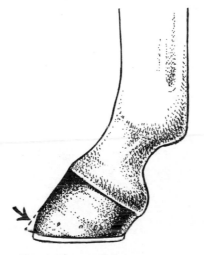

Dumped toe

Common Shoeing Problems

a. Improper leveling of the foot before shoeing. It is vital that the horse is walked and trotted on a level surface before being shod. Levelling with the foot held up often leads to improper balance with the ground.

b. Excessive burning of the foot when the horse is being hot-shod. The shoe must be made to fit the foot and not vice versa.

c. Excessive rasping of the wall in cold-shoeing, to make the foot fit the shoe.

d. Excessive rasping of the clenches, thereby weakening them.

e. Hammering clips against the wall may damage the pedal bone.

f. Excessive paring of the frog and sole. Only loose or overgrown portions should be removed.

g. Leaving the heels too high. Frog pressure must be maintained to avoid contraction of the foot.

h. Leaving the toes too long, thereby placing a strain on the structures at the back of the leg.

i. Pricking, or nailing too tight.

j. Reapplying shoes over bruised areas.

19 Physical Therapy

The purpose of any form of physical therapy is to foster the natural healing processes of the body. This is done in a number of ways from the simple application of heat and cold to massage and manipulation and the use of more complex equipment which has the same aim.

The purpose of applying heat is to dilate blood vessels and encourage blood flow into an area. The purpose of applying cold is the opposite — to constrict vessels and thus limit the extent of the body's reaction to injury. Heat is also applied in the form of poultices to draw infection from wounds etc. Cold is applied in laminitis as a means of reducing inflammation and controlling pain.

Faradic Therapy

This is used particularly for the diagnosis and treatment of muscular injuries. It has a vital place in modern horse medicine, and works on the principle of intermittent electric current applied to affected parts. This is achieved with two electrodes — a fixed pad and a moving head. The pad is placed in contact with the back of the patient and the head moved over the muscles to stimulate contraction and locate injuries. A suitable coupling medium (i.e. a gel which conducts the current into the tissues) must be used to allow contact.

The machine may operate on a single pole principle with the current travelling in one direction only. However more modern equipment allows for a bi-polar facility with the direction of the current being reversible. This permits a different therapeutic effect which has particular benefit for soft swellings and joint injuries.

While these machines are available for lay purchase it is important that the standard of application be such that there is no risk to the health of the animal. For this reason, it is vital that equine physiotherapy should become a regulated subject with appropriate training courses for those who wish to practise it.

Ultrasound

Ultra-high-frequency sound waves applied with an ultrasound machine can penetrate solid tissue to a depth of several inches. This is particularly beneficial in the treatment of injuries. The effect of the sound waves is to promote absorption of fluids, to stimulate circulation of deep parts and assist natural healing. Its effect on bone is largely beneficial, and it can be shown on x-ray that healing is encouraged in fractures of small bones and that remineralisation is in evidence in conditions such as pedal ostitis.

Some literature suggests that there is danger of demineralisation but there is no clinical support for this and the opposite is true in practice.

Risks of Ultrasound Use

a. Where infection is present there is a considerable danger that it may be spread to the general system causing septicaemia. Great care must be taken to ensure infection is not present before treatment is begun. If there is any doubt, withhold treatment.

b. Acute pain may be provoked in the early stages of inflammation and there is doubtful benefit in using ultrasound in the first day or two after more serious injury. Slight swellings may be treated earlier.

c. A coupling agent must be used and the head is moved constantly to prevent overheating of tissues.

d. Where pain is evoked on use, the machine should be turned to a pulsed-wave mode or the strength reduced. Pain will only be noted in the centre of the injury and it is wise to treat only the outer surrounds of the area initially.

e. Treatment should be limited to a period not longer than five minutes, though this may be done twice daily.

f. Ultrasound is of questionable help where there is haemorrhage, and could be counter-productive.

g. By removing the products of inflammation, ultrasound relieves pain and reduces heat. However it should be appreciated that this may leave an injured area at risk, e.g. tendons may appear to be perfect after treatment but will break down again if not rested until repair is complete. The same may apply to damaged joints and other structures — this effect is more marked with lasers.

Decisions on such matters are best made by experienced people who are qualified to do so. Removing the symptoms of inflammation can have its advantages but it can also expose an animal to further injury if the dangers are not properly understood.

Uses of Ultrasound

a. In any strain to a joint or its supporting ligaments.
b. As an adjunct to Faradic therapy on damaged muscles.
c. On tendons and ligaments to reduce inflammation. The limitations of therapy must be appreciated and the structure given adequate time to recover afterwards.
d. On noninfectious soft swellings, e.g. bursitis.
e. As an aid to the repair of small bone fractures, e.g. sesamoids. To relieve lameness in pedal ostitis.
f. Treatment of wounds, especially slow-healing wounds.
g. Control of proud flesh.
h. Physical injuries to the coronary band.

Lasers

Low-power infrared laser therapy is used for very similar conditions to those treated with ultrasound. It is more effective in its ability to reduce inflammation in certain situations, thereby increasing the danger of animals being returned to work too early. It has a marked effect in the reduction of pain, and is favoured for the treatment of sore shins of young racehorses.

Neither lasers nor ultrasound will return a chronically damaged muscle to full working use on their own. They will reduce pain and permit treated animals to be worked or raced. However there is unlikely to be a permanent cure without the use of Faradic treatment.

Pulsing Electromagnetic Fields

Although this equipment works on a different basis from lasers and ultrasound, its use is aimed at the same range of conditions, and different pads are supplied with the equipment to enable treatment of various parts of the body. Large pads for back treatment are available and these can be left on the animal, as can leg boots.

Magnets

These are being used increasingly to stimulate circulation in injured areas. They are available incorporated into special boots for various parts of the limbs. Small magnets are attached to the hoofs with success in some chronic conditions.

20 Stable Management

Good management is essential to disease control because bad management is a primary contributing cause of many diseases, infectious and otherwise. We have already referred to *azoturia*, also known as Monday Morning Disease, and noted the combined influence of management error and disease expression. The horse was given full rations on a rest day then taken out and worked as if there had been no change in his routine. The problem could have been avoided.

Management is, similarly, a key factor in modern infectious disease outbreaks and their spread. Workers can carry infection from one animal to another, physically, and from one yard to another if access is open to them. While this is hardly intentional it is, nevertheless, entirely feasible, so that hygiene is now a vital consideration in all dealings with large numbers of horses.

It is critical to consider every aspect of an animal's day, his exercise, feeding and stabling, in relation to the influence each can have on disease.

Points to Note

a. Is the horse normal when *first seen* in the morning? Has he eaten, and drunk his water? Is he happy and interested in your arrival? Is he moving freely about the stable?

b. Is anything abnormal seen when his rugs are removed — any galls from saddle, girth etc.? Any cough or nasal discharges?

c. Are his feet cold and shoes firmly attached and not bearing on the sole? Is the frog full and healthy?

d. When *ridden out* is he sound in action, moving freely and well?

e. *After exercise*, is he lame, blowing excessively or otherwise distressed? Has he sweated a great deal?
f. *Before returning* to the stable, brush the horse down or hose and dry his legs.
g. Are there any cuts or grazes, any sign of discomfort in the legs?
h. At *afternoon* or *evening stables*, has the horse eaten his feed and is he drinking water?
i. Is there any sign of illness, lameness, any heat in the legs or joints? Are droppings normal in texture and quantity? Is the horse staling normally?
j. Is the animal warm in his surroundings and free from any draughts, but not overwarm?

Aside from these observations, the person caring for an animal must evaluate the quality of hay and feed, and give care to bedding making sure it is clean and dry. Fouling of the air by urine or faeces acts as an irritant to the lining of the respiratory passages and this fosters infection. Keep bedding clean and dry at all times, never allowing dirt build-up because of bad stable drainage or poor floor design.

The quality of hay and straw is basic to the development and control of conditions such as COPD. Musty or mouldy hay can also cause digestive upsets in some animals fed on it, but the spores in poor quality hay or bedding can cause respiratory problems for almost all horses.

Stable Hygiene and Environment

a. Tack and grooming kits may facilitate spread of infection from one animal to another.
b. Hands, clothing, shoes and boots can carry infection.
c. Brushes, barrows and other implements may do likewise.
d. Muck and feed sacks are other sources of spread.
e. Organisms flourish on dirty buckets, feed and water bowls.
f. Limit dust disturbance in the animal's presence.
g. When judging the animal's warmth, do it objectively. Just because you are too warm from mucking out or grooming does not mean the animal is feeling the same.
h. Decisions on draught control should allow for weather changes which may occur in the night. A horse is in less danger of

infection when too warm than when too cold.

i. Wash regularly the sheaths of colts and geldings with warm water and mild soap.

Notes on Feeding

The following table shows the comparative values of different foods and gives an indication as to their choice in the class of work.

	Dry Matter %	Protein %	Oil %	Digestible Energy %	Fibre %
Hay	85	9.7	2.5	1.75	30
Oats	87	10	5	3	10
Barley	86	10	1.5	3.2	4.5
Maize	87	10	4	3.6	2.2
Bran	87	15	4	2.6	10
Beans	86	25	1.5	3.2	7
Linseed	92	24	36	5.8	5

As an addendum to the above, consider:

a. Hay by itself is variable in quality and food value. It is subject to variation from the type of grasses involved, from the condition it was in when cut, from the weather when saved, and from the manner in which it was stored. However, because of being low in energy and high in fibre, hay alone is not adequate for hard or fast work.

b. Oats, being a good source of starch and protein, are well suited to the needs of the working horse — depending of course on the quality of the oats. They are readily digested and not too bulky. Although the modern trend is for higher levels, the amount of protein in oats is an ideal basis for a racing diet; horses have raced successfully on it for generations. There is little proof that higher protein improves performance.

c. Barley is used, very often boiled, as a minor dietary source of carbohydrate. However, it has a tendency to be heating and to create digestive disturbances in Thoroughbreds. Some horses tend to tie-up under its influence. Hunters and ponies digest it more easily.

d. Maize is not a suitable sole feed for horses, though it is added in small quantities to many modern mixes.

e. Bran is high in phosphorus, which can be a complicating factor if fed in excess to young animals. It is a useful laxative, and may be added in small proportions to oats in a mixed diet.

f. Various types of bean are added to modern rations. They are high in protein and are useful for raising the protein level in diets which are otherwise inadequate. But care needs to be taken in their introduction and not to feed them at too high a level in the ration.

g. Linseed is fed as a laxative to fit horses, once weekly, normally boiled or in oil form. It has proven benefits for sick and unthrifty horses, and it gives a bloom to the coat.

To raise the protein level of a low value diet any of the following may be added:

	Protein
Grass meal	17%
Brewer's grain	25%
Fishmeal	70%
Linseed meal	35%
Meat and bone meal	48%
Skim milk – dried	35%
Soya bean	47%

However, it must be appreciated that any addition of high-protein sources has to be intelligently applied. The idea is only to add sufficient to bring the existing diet up to a specified level. Also, the quality of the protein in these feeds varies. Soya bean meal is a popular source of protein for increasing the level in concentrate rations. It is slightly irritant when first given and should be introduced at a low percentage in the diet.

The recommended protein levels in feeds for horses of different ages on a maintenance diet of grass or good hay are:

Foal – at weaning	16%–18%
Yearling	14%–16%
Two-year-old in training	12%–14%
Mature horse in training	12%–14%
Broodmare in foal	10%–12%
Broodmare lactating	12%–14%

Many trainers are feeding concentrates at protein levels well above those recommended here. Twelve per cent is probably adequate, if not ideal, for most mature horses in training. With disease conditions involving the liver, feeding higher levels of protein can delay recovery of form. Inevitably, decisions to feed high levels have to be weighed against the workload and the ability of the animal to hold condition and performance. While it is not possible to specify absolute guidelines for individual animals, the best advice is to feed with caution. Increase feed levels gradually with work. Increase protein levels when demand calls for it, as long as there is not another problem causing the animal to lose condition.

Quantities fed have to reflect the size and age of the horse, his workload, appetite, condition, etc.

Check points

a. Sudden changes in the feeding routine are a danger to an animal's health. Change over gradually using hay and light mashes as an introduction from grass to solid feeding.
b. Do not suddenly change from solid feeding to grass either, or turn animals from very poor to lush grazing too quickly.
c. Purge or physic horses in work at least once annually. Feed only hay and water until the purgative has had its full effect and gradually return to normal feeding afterwards. Ideally, this is done when the animal first comes in. As long as the dose of purgative is controlled the animal can return to gradual work as soon as its effects are over.
d. Feeding is still an art – even if time does not always allow for its practice now – and the eye of the feeder is critical to establishing the individual needs of any animal. The quality

of food is the choice of the feeder, and a judgement has to be made on whether the quantity fed allows the animal to do the work demanded and hold his condition. Such a wide variety of manufactured feeds are now used that manufacturers guidelines are necessary information on feeding levels.

e. Do not use too high a protein ration. Twelve per cent protein is an adequate level for any mature animal. The feeding of too high a level can lead to fat deposition and place a strain on metabolism.

f. Keep feeding simple — horses raced as successfully on oats and simple additives as they are now doing with so much variety in their diet.

g. Complex diets lead to inflammation of the bowel, ulcers and colic.

h. Monitor water intake and always cater for electrolyte shortage. Water quality is as important to the horse as to the human.

i. Never feed an animal solely on bran. Bran is high in phosphorus and can cause bone disorders.

j. Feed clean, nourishing, top quality hay to horses in work. Bad hay will not only have a low feed value it will promote fermentation and carry spores to provoke COPD.

k. Remember barley does not suit all horses. It is important to be observant and be prepared to change a diet if it is causing problems.

l. The regular use of linseed as the basis for a mash is good practice for those with the time to spare. This can be prepared by adding a cupful of linseed to a gallon of water and simmering it for 6–8 hours. Strain through muslin, and the jelly produced will be adequate for two horses mixed in a mash.

m. Remember the need for organic-food quality. Horses do best when kept clear of many of the contaminants found as a result of modern farming. Sprays and chemicals can be toxic to the liver and certain fertilisers are thought to influence adversely the absorption of minerals such as calcium, phosphorus, magnesium, manganese, copper, etc.

n. Do not give more than one mineral supplement without advice from an expert. It is possible to cause toxicity by overfeeding numerous elements.

Appetite

Most horses will eat if treated as individuals, and if allowed some variety in their feed. Poor feeders may be suffering from dehydration, infection or even indigestion. Solving these problems will enhance their appetite.

Do not present a horse with one huge feed. If it is necessary to get large amounts into an animal on full work, divide the feeds and spread them throughout the day.

Do not feed before work. Allow at least an hour to elapse, or, alternatively, feed when the horse comes in.

Chaff added to feed will encourage animals that bolt their food to chew properly.

Horses should have water available to them at all times, though automatic drinking bowls make it difficult to gauge consumption.

Exercise

It is important to build up fitness steadily over a period of time. Health is the first priority for working horses and it is vital that simple problems such as worm burdens, low-grade infections, etc., be eliminated before an animal goes into a training prgramme.

Early exercise at the walk and trot must allow for the horse's unfit state, but it is also important that the animal finds his exercise demanding. Horses arriving home from exercise too fresh may well require more time out.

Encourage the animal to walk briskly and use himself when ridden; when he is coping well with this he should begin trotting. Do not proceed to cantering until the horse is able to trot strongly for extended periods on rising ground. A great many horses suffer muscular damage through cantering too early, or through being asked for too much speed when not ready to give it.

Full fitness takes considerable time to achieve − longer than is normally allowed today − so each step should be taken with care. While animals will continue to get fit through their training programme, injury is more likely before full fitness is attained.

Clipping

Horses are clipped when their coats grow too long while in training. It helps to reduce sweating and loss of body fluids. It also makes grooming simpler and drying off more manageable.

The loss of the coat needs to be compensated for with extra clothing while the animal is stabled.

Bedding

Good wheat straw has always been favoured as bedding for horses, as long as it is clean and dust free. Barley and oat straw have also been used. However, if the straw is of too high a quality, the animals may eat it and this can cause problems with their diet. Too much roughage is likely to cause fermentation, which will increase the bulk of the bowel and interfere with work.

Shavings and sawdust provide a dry, warm bed which is free from spores. Peat is used for the same reason but is not as clean. These types of bedding are usually kept in a deep-litter system, with dirt and wet being removed twice daily and the bed freshened with some clean material added to the top.

Shredded paper is fashionable, especially for horses with wind problems, but, as with any deep-litter system, it has its advantages and disadvantages. Paper is spore-free, and relatively free of dust, however, when fresh, it is light of body and does not provide much cushioning until a deep-litter system is established.

The disadvantage of any deep-litter system is the build up of moisture beneath the animal, and the adverse effect this may have on humidity, warmth and hygiene. Horses invariably appear more comfortable and relax better when bedded on good, clean straw.

Vices

Weaving

A weaver is a horse which, when at rest, swings his head methodically from side to side, usually shifting his weight from one foreleg to the other at the same time.

This problem is an expression of nervousness or boredom and is commonly seen in stabled animals. Some horses weave only when standing with their head over a half door, others weave when anticipating food, and some horses will weave for a short time when moved to a new home and then stop doing it. Confirmed cases weave anywhere; once the habit has been acquired it is hard to stop. Others may develop the vice from watching it enacted.

While it was formerly considered to be a source of weight loss and hence poor performance in competing horses, a less serious view of the problem is taken today. Many good racehorses weave at times and are not affected by it. However, the problem is still a vice which must be declared when an animal is presented for sale, failing which he can be returned to his vendor.

Various devices have been used to control weaving, including anti-weaving bars or grills on stable doors, but, although they lessen the problem, they do not eliminate it.

Wind-sucking and Crib-biting

A wind-sucker will grab at fixed objects such as sills and doors with his teeth, then swallow air while arching his neck and making a pronounced grunting noise. A crib-biter grabs and eats wooden fixtures but may not swallow air.

These are serious habits which, once contracted, do not tend to be forgotten, and both conditions have to be declared when horses are presented for sale.

Crib-biters are often found to have undue wear of the incisor teeth. Therefore, when buying a horse, worn incisors should make the buyer suspect that the horse is in fact a crib-biter.

Various devices have been used to prevent horses from swallowing wind and the one shown in the accompanying diagram is by far the most popular.

A number of surgical operations have been used for this condition with varying degrees of success.

21 Care and Management of the Broodmare and Foal

While it is essentially true that nature looks after the mare through the often explosive experience of foaling, the value of a foal today, and knowledge of the mishaps which may occur, favour the idea of full supervision at the time of birth. Also, the delicate nature of the foal during the first hours of his life means that help should always be at hand in case it is needed.

Foaling units and stations are a feature of today's Thoroughbred breeding programmes and both mare and foal are monitored at every stage from birth onwards. The same risks exist for non-thoroughbreds too and it is always regrettable when either a foal or mare — whatever their value — are lost through lack of supervision.

Foaling can be a traumatic event, particularly for very anxious mares. The strength of their contractions can cause great damage to both themselves and their foals, even to the point of death. A percentage of mares do considerable damage to the soft tissues of the cervix, vagina, vulva and rectum through impatience. This damage can take a long time to repair, and can be the cause of the mare not getting in foal again.

The Reproductive System

The ovaries of the mare are attached to the roof of the abdomen just in front of the pelvis, they connect with the horns of the uterus along the Fallopian tubes. It is along this path that the ovum travels and meets the semen which is deposited through the cervix and into the bed of the uterus.

The cervix is placed at the junction of the vagina and uterus and its purpose is to close the uterus off from the exterior except during oestrus and foaling. It is a soft structure when open which permits the discharge of accumulated secretions — including those related to in-

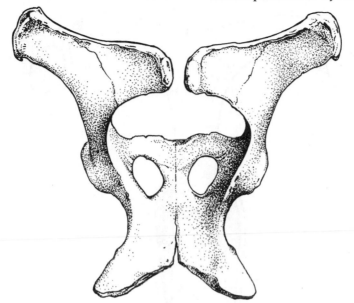

The pelvis of the horse from behind

fection. When closed, its part in the maintenance of pregnancy is critical. It is then small and tight, impenetrable to organisms. Any tearing of the cervix can have a limiting effect on the mare's chances of holding on to a conceptus.

The vulva is important as the external control of entry of organisms into the reproductive system. When it is deficient, as is common in Thoroughbreds, infection of the vagina ensues and the condition may be marked by a tendency to suck air. This problem is treated surgically and the lips of the vulva are sutured together.

The normal *breeding season* for mares is, to an extent, grass related, though light is a factor and oestrus periods can occur as early as January in mild weather conditions. With horses other than Thoroughbreds, it is generally planned to have foals arrive when there is grass in abundance to help the mare with her milk. For Thoroughbreds, with their January 1st birth date, the earlier the foal the greater his value as a two-year-old racing prospect. For this reason, barren and maiden mares are frequently kept under lights in the early months of the year in order to encourage them to come into season early. The advent of grass still has a great influence on the situation.

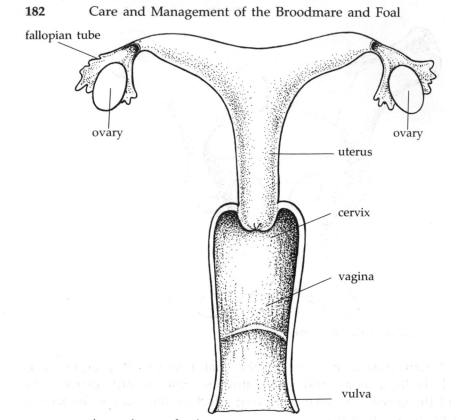

A mare's reproductive organs

While opinions differ, the usually accepted *length* of a mare's *cycle* — with room for considerable variation — is 21 days between ovulations. The length of the heat period varies with the season; it can be very extended in the early months of the year and shorten to about four to six days when the main flush of grass arrives and the days get longer and warmer. Ovulation usually occurs about 24 hours before the end of heat.

Mating is a potential source of infection for the mare, and the delicate tissues of the vagina and cervix are commonly bruised at the time. It is modern stud practice to limit the covering of mares to once per heat period if possible, closely related to the time of ovulation.

Stallion semen is viable for at least 48 hours, except in horses with fertility problems. Mares are not the most prolific breeders and there is a substantial *loss of early conceptions* on average.

The *gestation period* — length of pregnancy — is in the region of 340 days, though there is wide variation between individual mares.

The *signs of oestrus* are easy to recognise and are best detected in the presence of a teaser or stallion.

   a. The mare will be extremely aggressive if not in season, and any sign of acceptance of the teaser's approach is likely to be significant.
   b. The degree of acceptance will vary with the animal and the stage of the cycle.
   c. When close to ovulation the mare will usually accept mounting and present herself for covering by raising the tail and everting the clitoris. Urine may be released.

When in season the mare has a cervical swab taken to check for bacterial infection of the uterus. Swabs for *contagious equine metritis* are taken, as recommended in the controls mentioned earlier. While positive swabs are rare now, prevention is critical to the international transportation of mares and stallions.

If there is any indication that the mare is a *vaginal wind sucker*, the vulva is stitched to control the problem.

Mares are *covered* with varying degrees of *control* applied to save the stallion from being kicked. A twitch and anti-kicking boots are common, while some stud managers will also have a foreleg strapped up. Some use hobbles or more severe forms of restraint. Many modern studs are less fearful of hurting the stallion as long as the mare is teased well and found receptive. Too severe restraint can often lead to accidents. Mares which will not stand are very often not properly in season and need careful internal examination by an experienced person to detect the cause.

The mare is *scanned* at about 16 days for pregnancy using an ultrasonic scanner. Detected pregnancies are carefully examined for evidence of twinning, and watched for progressive development of the foal over a period of time. *Twin pregnancies* are dealt with manually and there is a high percentage of success in removing one and allowing the other to develop. It is rare for a mare to give birth to two healthy offspring in a twin birth, or even to carry twins for the full term.

Mares found not to be in foal will be *teased* until they either come into season again voluntarily or are induced with prostaglandin.

Stallions are kept indoors during the stud season. They are exercised by riding or lungeing to keep them fit for their work, and this is vital to their fertility. They are turned out to grass during the day in the closed season.

Foaling

  a. Solid feeding should be given throughout pregnancy to encourage normal development of the foal and to prepare the mare for lactation.

  b. Foaling boxes should be of an adequate size to accommodate the mare and allow her plenty of room to lie down. There should also be plenty of room in which to give assistance.

  c. A light is left on permanently so that the mare can be observed without disturbing her.

  d. A source of clean hot water should be available, as well as disinfectant and lubricant. Care must be taken to avoid the introduction of infection into the vagina by helpers.

  e. Mares are best left unshod to prevent any injury to the foal.

  f. Ensure that mares with stitched vulvas have the stitches removed before foaling.

Signs of Imminent Foaling

  a. Full udder development with the teats fully everted.

  b. Slackness of the muscles to either side of the base of the tail.

  c. Relaxation and swelling of the vulva.

  d. Extrusion of wax from the teats, perhaps with some milk running.

  e. The mare may walk her box and show signs of unease.

  f. Sweating.

  g. The mare will usually lie down for the beginning of labour and as foetal membranes begin to show.

Foaling will normally follow quickly after this point with the foal's hooves showing first followed by the front of the head. The whole process is over in a matter of fifteen or twenty minutes. If no signs are seen once the mare has started forcing, professional help must be provided quickly.

Points to Note

a. There is little time for delay with a foaling mare. If a foal's leg is back and can be found easily, bring it forward gently.

b. If the foal is caught at the hips a gentle pull may be applied to assist release.

c. Remove any membrane which remains over the foal's head to prevent suffocation.

d. Leave the foal attached to the mother to allow the complete passage of blood into the foal's circulation before separation. It is wise to stand back and not interfere while this is happening. Mares which get up too quickly and break the cord deprive the foal of vital pints of blood.

e. If the foal is not breathing regularly, clear any mucus blocking the nasal passages. Breathing may be stimulated by gentle pressure over the ribs and lungs.

f. Dress the navel cord with iodine solution once the mare has separated. This will help to prevent joint-ill. Do not tie the cord except with expert advice or to prevent impending herniation.

g. The foal is routinely injected with antibiotics and tetanus antitoxin as a preventive measure. Most major studs follow this practice and find it effective.

h. Colt foals are given phosphate enemas immediately after birth to lessen the problem of retained meconium; colts having a greater problem with this than fillies.

i. Where there is a danger of lowered immunity — perhaps due to the mare having *run milk* (lost milk prior to the foal's birth) — the foal is given plasma intravenously.

j. The foal should be encouraged to suck within an hour of birth. If, for any reason, this is not possible, some milk should be drawn from the mare and given by bottle. This ensures that the foal gets the full benefit of colostrum (the first milk containing the protective antibodies) and the nourishment can help to revive a weak foal.

k. If the mare retains her placenta, veterinary assistance may be required to remove it. It should not be left more than 12 hours, and the vet should be called earlier if she shows any sign of being off colour.

l. Care must be taken to observe whether or not the mare accepts her offspring. Some mares refuse to have anything to do with the foal from the start. In bad cases the foal may have to be taken away at an early stage and fostered. In other cases vigilance is needed for the first few days until the mare gradually settles down and accepts him. The foal may need to be protected, perhaps kept away from the mare and only brought in for feeding. Many bad cases work out successfully, and even mares who initially objected strongly to their foal will, on occasion, relent.

m. The mare and foal can be moved from the foaling box once the foal has adjusted to his new environment, and can be given an hour at grass after a few days.

n. The mare will come into season at any time from about five to 12 days after foaling. Traditionally, the foaling heat was said to occur at nine days, but the timing varies widely. It is a short-heat period − lasting 1−3 days − and fertile in young mares. If there were no complications at foaling and the womb has returned to its normal size, the mare is covered.

o. Foals often scour while the mare is in heat. This is controlled by limiting milk intake. Various remedies also exist, but, if the scour persists and the foal stops suckling, professional help is needed.

p. The foal is weaned in the autumn of the year. This is done in various ways, and the mare and foal should be kept apart after weaning.

q. Orphan foals are successfully reared by foster mothers. If none is available, artificial feeding is simplified today with the availability of milk-replacer and special pelleted feeds. Introduce the foal slowly to new feed and do not be tempted to overfeed.

Castration

Colts are cut either as foals in the autumn or as yearlings in the spring of the following year. The operation is often done with the foal standing, under local anaesthetic and sedation, and the animal is then turned out to grass immediately afterwards. The operation is not performed during bad weather or heavy frosts to avoid infection of the castration site. Tetanus antiserum is given.

Diseases of Foals

Retention of the Meconium

Meconium is the accumulated faecal material in the foal's bowel at birth. It is usually hard and lumpy and is passed in the first hours of life. Colts tend to have greater trouble with meconium than fillies because of the size of a colt's pelvis, and for this reason most Thoroughbred colt foals are given a phosphate enema at birth. This preventive is usually adequate though, on occasion, there are more troublesome cases.

Symptoms: The foal will show signs of unease and pain. This can vary from simple discomfort to extreme pain with sweating. It strains and forces continually. In serious cases it may stop sucking.

Diagnosis: Forcing, in the first hours, is marked. On examination of the rectum with a lubricated, gloved finger, a pellet of meconium will be felt impacted into the pelvic entrance. This is not a job for an amateur as the rectum can easily be punctured by sharp fingernails and rough handling.

Treatment: Gentleness is important in dealing with any young foal, and there is a limit to the amount of handling that can be done to the delicate rectum. If an enema has been given and the foal is still forcing, liquid paraffin should be given by stomach tube and a further phosphate enema administered. Most cases respond well, particularly as the lubricant effect of the colostrum also helps to remove meconium.

It may be necessary to sedate foals which have very acute pain but this decision will have to be made by the attending veterinary surgeon.

One of the dangers with this condition is that it can give rise to rupture of the bladder, which is a very serious complication. The problem should never be ignored in the hope it will pass off.

Surgery is required in very obstinate cases.

Diarrhoea or Scouring

A distinction needs to be made between noninfectious scours — which may occur when a foal is getting too much milk, or during the foaling heat — and infection. With noninfectious causes, scour is controlled by limiting the foal's intake of milk. This can be done with a muzzle which is removed periodically. If the condition gets worse or the temperature rises, professional help is needed. The foal may need antibiotic treatment and steps to limit fluid loss and replace lost electrolytes.

Symptoms: The consistency of the faeces changes from the very hard, dark pellets of meconium to the softer, milk-tinged droppings which appear in the first couple of days. When this becomes watery and strong-smelling the condition is in need of attention. Any temperature has to be taken seriously. The foal may stop sucking and become drowsy and tend to lie down. Some will drink water excessively.

Diagnosis: The distinction between normality and serious disease is made on the basis of the foal's behaviour, his inclination to suck, his temperature and the degree of scouring.

Scouring caused by infection in the first days of life may indicate a failure of the foal's immunity, or, alternatively, the presence of a virulent organism in the foaling area. Swabs may help to identify the organism and pinpoint a suitable antibiotic.

Treatment: Antibiotics for initial treatment will have to be selected on the basis of the severity of the condition. Salmonella infection is an especially serious problem marked by very high temperatures and depression of the foal. There is quick dehydration and a high percentage of foals die with the disease.

Replacement of lost fluid may be accomplished by stomach tube or intravenously in acute cases. Plasma may be of benefit.

Drugs such as kaolin may be of help in soothing the inflamed bowel and controlling fluid loss.

Navel-ill or Joint-ill

This condition usually appears in the first week of life. It occurs when infection gains access to the bloodstream, mainly through the navel.

Symptoms: The foal becomes dull and listless and is found to have a temperature. It is slow to suck. There may be swelling in one or more joints, or the navel itself may be hot and swollen.

Diagnosis: In the absence of any enlarged joints the condition is diagnosed on signs of systemic infection and local infection on the navel. Swollen joints must not be confused with those caused through physical injury.

Treatment: As the condition may reflect a lowered immune status, steps are taken to counter this by giving the foal plasma. Antibiotics are used intensively to counter systemic infection. Joint swellings, once they become evident, are an unwelcome sign as the condition is then difficult to reverse.

Prevention: Cleanliness of the foaling environment is critical. It is also important that the broken navel cord is immersed in iodine solution and that it is not contaminated by ligatures or implements which are not sterile. An antibiotic spray applied to the stump will only kill the organisms which are susceptible to it. Antibiotic injections at birth are a definite preventive help.

Care must be taken about milk intake and its quality. If the mare has run milk for any time before foaling and the colostrum has lost its clear, thick consistency, colostrum from another mare should be given — if this is available — within the first hours after birth. The foal should be assisted with a bottle if unable to suck.

Sleepy-foal Disease

This is an infectious condition which is marked by extreme dullness and death in a high percentage of affected foals. It is rare nowadays because of the routine use of antibiotics at birth.

Barkers and Dummies

These conditions are relatively common, and are seen in the first 48 hours of life. The cause is best explained by the technical name — neonatal maladjustment syndrome.

Symptoms: The foal appears to walk into objects, as if he were blind. He generally goes off suck or sucks without normal vigour. He may continually walk the box and press his head into walls, etc. Some foals are unable to stand and may thrash about and go into convulsions.

Diagnosis: There is no temperature and no sign of infection. Some foals appear dull and incoordinate while others are only slightly affected.

Treatment: Many milder cases recover when fed by stomach tube. This should be done every four hours, until the foal returns to normal. Some improve dramatically with a single feed.

Foals with more advanced symptoms require drugs to control convulsions and need to be kept in a stable, warm environment.

Jaundice of Foals

This is similar to human rhesus factor jaundice and is caused by incompatibility in the blood of sire and dam. It only occurs after the foal has sucked from its dam, the illness being due to interreaction between the foal's red blood cells and the absorbed milk.

Symptoms: Depending on the degree of incompatibility, symptoms may appear in the first 24 hours of life, or later. The foal is dull and listless, and jaundice is seen at an early stage in the membranes of the eyes, nostrils and mouth. The urine may have a darkened colour.

Diagnosis: The jaundice must not be confused with the discolouration of membranes which occurs in some infectious conditions, such as herpes virus infection. The onset of illness is related to the intake of milk.

Treatment: Replacement transfusion is the only hope in advanced cases, and the prognosis with these is not good.

Prevention: Cross-matching of foal's blood with mare's milk can usually be arranged at any modern stud. In suspect cases the foal is given colostrum from another mare and kept away from his own mother's milk for the first 24 hours. After this time it is normally safe to commence normal suckling. The mare will have been milked out during the first day.

Pneumonia in Foals

Pneumonia may result from a number of causes and is frequently a result of poor foal immunity.

Symptoms: The disease is unusual in the first days of life, except where there is an immune deficiency, or in herpes virus infections. The temperature rises and the foal will be depressed with an increased respiratory rate and may be sweating.

Diagnosis: The deepened breathing is marked and the associated rise in temperature may be accompanied by a nasal discharge and coughing.

In some cases the organism causing the condition may be very resistant and will need to be identified by culturing infected material.

Treatment: Immediate antibiotic therapy is carried out, and resistant cases will require sensitivity tests.

In Rhodococcus infection there is a tendency to abscess formation in the lungs and this can lengthen greatly the period of treatment and darken the prognosis.

The Importance of Colostrum

Colostrum is vital not only for nourishing the newborn foal but also for providing antibodies for protection from infections the mare will have encountered through life. The foal's immune system is not developed at birth and he relies on his mother's transferred protection. Colostrum also helps to lubricate meconium and expel it.

Vital antibodies are only contained in the colostrum for a limited time after foaling and the foal is only able to absorb them from his bowel during the early hours of life. These periods vary from animal to animal and may be as short as a few hours or as long as a full day. Therefore, good management dictates that the foal be given full protection as early as possible.

Colostrum may have lost its value where a mare has run milk before foaling. It may also be defective for other reasons which are not fully understood. If it is suspected that a foal has not been adequately protected, plasma from the mother is a simple effective way of transferring the same immunity.

Contracted Tendons in Newborn Foals

Contraction of the flexor tendons is a congenital condition which may result from placement in the womb. It may also have nutritional or genetic causes.

Symptoms: The foal's front legs are most commonly affected. The severity of the contraction varies from an upright stance to one where the foal is unable to straighten his legs and attempts to stand on the front of his fetlocks.

Diagnosis: The condition is mechanical and there is no associated infection.

Treatment: Less severe cases will usually correct themselves without treatment. Where contraction is marked the legs may be placed in plaster casts, or surgery may be needed in extreme cases.

22 Nursing the Sick Animal and First Aid

Nursing

The purpose of sick care is to foster the natural repair and defensive processes of the body. The following principles apply:

a. The maintenance of body temperature. We do this by dressing the animal in rugs and by providing an atmosphere which is warm, dry and stable.

   Artificial heat is provided on occasion by infrared overhead, or wall, heaters when an animal is excessively cold or in shock.

b. Feeding the sick animal is a vital part of any nursing programme.

   When horses are completely off food and water, intravenous fluids are given to maintain life and counter dehydration. Up to 40 litres per day may be required for a sick adult animal. Electrolytes and amino-acid mixtures are commonly added until the animal has resumed eating.

   When the horse is able to drink, electrolytes are added to the drinking water. Appetite is tempted with fresh grass or warm mashes.

c. Fresh air is a necessity for all sick animals, but its provision must be tempered with common sense. Draughts are caused by overventilation, by creating cross-flows, and by failing to understand what the horse needs. Their influence on the respiratory system is swift and damaging; resistance is lowered giving infection a greater chance.

   Air extraction, if unsatisfactory, has to be arranged discretely and without lowering body defences.

d. Cleanliness and hygiene are important in nursing. If an animal is suffering from an infectious condition, steps must be taken to ensure the problem is not spread. It is important also to ensure that infection is not introduced to a recuperating animal while it is susceptible to attack.

e. Beds are kept dry and clean and tended regularly.

f. Dust is minimised – no dusty hay or straw shaken up in the animal's stable.

g. Exercise is started as soon as possible, even if this only amounts to a walk about the box or yard. Gradually, the exercise is increased.

h. When the appetite improves the animal is fed to restore lost weight, but care is taken to avoid overfeeding or to give food which is binding or indigestible.

i. Temperature, pulse and respiration are checked and recorded every 12 hours.

j. Evident discharges are washed away as they accumulate.

k. Turn recumbent animals every couple of hours to prevent bedsores.

l. When poulticing infections, replace every 12 hours initially, and apply as warm as the hand can bear it.

m. Let air get at wounds after a few days as some infections proliferate under cover.

First Aid

a. Wounds which occur while hunting or racing are dressed with clean bandaging and gauze until they can be dealt with fully.

b. Physical injuries – including fractures – to the lower legs are strongly supported, usually bandaging both legs at the same time to save strain on the sound leg. Pain-killers may be required and a veterinary surgeon will administer them after examining the animal.

c. The injured animal is made comfortable for transport home. A drink of water and bite of hay may help to take his mind off the pain.

d. Slings may have to be provided for animals with badly injured legs, or paralysis from herpes infection. While these can be roughly constructed, all points of contact must be well padded and the animal protected from contact sores and from doing damage to himself in his surroundings.

e. Stop bleeding by applying pressure locally. A bandage or ligature may be applied, but must be slackened as soon as the bleeding is controlled to permit blood circulation in healthy tissues.

f. Tetanus protection for wounds is critical. Unvaccinated horses are given antiserum when at risk.

g. Keep colicy horses on their feet and moving until help arrives. Do not allow them to throw themselves about or roll.

h. With eye injuries, clean with warm boric solution. If in doubt about the extent of the injury seek professional help.

i. Tie choking animals away from food and water.

j. Reduce inflammation of injured tendons with cold applications and support.

k. Horses with acute laminitis may get relief from cold hosing or by being stood in a stream.

l. Submerge feet which have been pricked or punctured into a strong antiseptic solution before poulticing.

m. Horses with azoturia are moved gently, if possible, or else have to be boxed home.

n. Oxygen is given by inhalation to horses which suffer from acute insufficiency after racing.

o. Electrolytes are given orally or intravenously to horses suffering from exhaustion after long-distance rides. Cool down with cold water if required.

Throughout this book further advice has been given on first-aid requirements for specific conditions.

Administration of Drugs

Injection is *subcutaneous* when a drug is deposited under the skin. *Intramuscular* injection places the drug in muscle tissue. *Intravenous* injections go directly into the blood stream through a vein. It is important to know that not all drugs can be given into a vein — it is possible to kill an animal with drugs administered the wrong way. Drugs intended to be given intravenously may be irritant when placed under the skin.

The veterinary surgeon will decide on the best way to use the drugs chosen. If he/she wants to establish high blood levels quickly, injection is given into the vein. On the contrary, if it is required to delay the time the active drug is released, the intramuscular route may be selected. Drugs like anabolic steroids are given in an oily base into muscle. In this way active drug is released into the system over a delayed period of time, thus having a longer effect.

It is important when giving injections to horses to be 100 per cent sterile at every step taken. The skin must be swabbed with surgical spirit; needles and syringes − mostly disposable today − should be new and be taken directly from their sterile containers. Care must be taken not to contaminate either site or instrument with unclean hands or by bringing them into contact with any surface matter.

Ideally there should be no reaction after injection. This depends not only on the substance being injected but also on the technique of the individual doing it. To be rough is to damage tissue and create an inflammatory reaction. It is important to remember that horses rely on their muscular system to perform. Damaged muscles − even from this source − are painful and do not function properly. Abscesses in deep muscle sites are likely after faulty injection techniques, therefore, where possible, avoid injecting into muscle bodies. Subcutaneous injections are simpler to give and less likely to provoke reaction. Intravenous injection is the most efficient and clean way to administer drugs − as long as they are recommended for use in this way by the manufacturer. Many drugs *cannot* be given into the vein. Some are too irritant for subcutaneous use.

Always follow the manufacturer's instructions and take the advice of your veterinary surgeon before administering injections to your horse.

Some drugs are given *by mouth* either for local affect on the bowel or their systemic effect when absorbed.

Many drugs are applied locally to the skin, eyes, nostrils, etc.

Antibiotics

These are drugs which, as their name implies, are designed to kill infectious organisms. As they are all controlled by law, their availability is restricted to strictly professional channels. The purpose of this is to prevent abuse by indiscriminate use and to protect the importance of these drugs to human medicine.

While different antibiotics act in different ways – and on different organisms – the individual veterinary surgeon's choice of drug will be dictated by the symptoms seen and the diagnosis made. Where the response is not satisfactory, further drugs will be selected on the basis of sensitivity tests.

Treatment with antibiotics is normally continued until the infection is fully controlled and the risk of resistant organisms taking over is eliminated. Treatment may be local – as in infected wounds – or systemic, when the drug is injected into the body.

Varieties

a. Penicillin. This was the first antibiotic discovered and it still has considerable use today.

   Its principal use in equine practice is in injectable form. It is, preferably, used intravenously in the soluble crystalline form. Suspended penicillin cannot be used in the vein and is given intramuscularly. This is the drug given for tetanus.

b. Ampicillin is a semi-synthetic drug closely related to penicillin. It has a broader spectrum of effect and also has the advantage of being able to be used orally.

c. Streptomycin is an antibiotic often used in combination with penicillin to cover a broader range of organisms. These drugs have been given extensively to foals at birth to prevent navel-ill and sleepy-foal disease. There is little danger of toxicity with them.

d. Neomycin is used for infections where its effectiveness is indicated by sensitivity tests. There is a slight danger of toxicity which is balanced against the risk to the patient of the infection suffered.

e. Oxytetracycline is a useful broad-spectrum antibiotic used in certain specific infections of horses, and where indicated by sensitivity test. There is a danger of bowel disturbance with this drug, but, again, this has to be weighed against the merits of the case.

f. Potentiated sulphonamides are very popular at present as a nontoxic, broad-spectrum antibiotic which can be given

either orally or by injection.
g. There is a very wide variety of other antibiotics in use.

Anthelminthics

These are worm doses for oral use and their selection should be based
on the type of worm and effectiveness of the drug. All information is
available from the manufacturer's literature.

Anti-inflammatory Drugs

As their name implies, these drugs are used to control inflammation.
Their availability is restricted and the decision to use them is left in
professional hands.

Cortisone and related drugs are used locally and by injection. Their
choice in therapy must depend on expert opinion as there are dangers
in their use and their anti-inflammatory nature creates a risk of infection.

Butazolidin is used extensively for relief of inflammation and pain in
injured horses. It can be given either orally or by injection and is
relatively nontoxic if continued over a long period in adult animals. It
has proved more toxic in foals and ponies. Drugs such as meclofenamic
acid are preferred for these animals because of lower toxicity.

Anabolic Steroids

These are synthetic male hormone derivatives used clinically for their
ability to promote tissue repair and stimulate recovery in convalescent
animals. They have a positive effect on certain aspects of metabolism.

It is unfortunate that anabolic steroids have been used unscrupulously
for their ability to promote muscle growth and enhance performance
in racing animals. They are important drugs in the treatment of sick animals and their availability must not be endangered by the dishonest few.

Anaesthetics, Sedatives and Analgesics

Local anaesthetics are used for tissue infiltration or surface deadening —
for the eyes, membranes and skin. Injectable forms are used for procedures such as stitching, nerve-blocking, and minor surgical procedures.

General anaesthetics are given either by intravenous injection or by inhalation. The administration of these drugs is a highly complex matter and is generally carried out by individuals with specialised training.

Sedatives are used for restraint in order to permit minor procedures to be carried out on fractious animals. There is a wide range of drugs available, the most commonly used of which is probably acetylpromazine. This drug is also a useful antispasmodic for the treatment of certain types of colic.

Analgesics, or pain killers, are used when indicated by a veterinary surgeon.

All drugs in this section are potentially dangerous and not available to the public.

Hormones

These are mostly synthetic drugs which duplicate natural body hormones and are used for a variety of purposes.

Oestrogen is the female hormone which is associated with development and release of the ovum. Its influence is wide and involves the preparation of the female tract for mating. It plays a critical part in the control of uterine infection.

Progesterone is vital to the events after the mare has ovulated. Its function is to maintain pregnancy and prevents the mare from coming back into season.

Prostaglandin is a synthetic hormone with the ability to bring mares into season by removing the corpus luteum. The ensuing oestrus occurs at anything from 12 hours to several days.

Luteinising hormone helps to promote ovulation when the mare has a ripe follicle and is close to natural ovulation.

Follicle-stimulating hormone helps the maturation of existing follicles, but is not widely used in modern stud practice.

Oxytocin causes contraction of the uterus and is mostly used to assist foaling or to reduce the size of the uterus afterwards.

Drugs Acting on the Respiratory System

There is a whole range of drugs available which have positive influences on the respiratory system. Many of these are used in conditions such as

COPD and in low-grade respiratory infections where it is desired to increase clearance from the tract.

Clenbuterol hydrochloride is used with considerable effect in allergic conditions, such as COPD. As long as the animal is removed from the cause of his allergy, the drug helps to relieve spasm of the bronchi and fosters muco-ciliary clearance.

Sodium cromoglycate is used as an inhalation to prevent the development of allergic respiratory disease.

Drugs Acting on the Kidneys

Frusemide is a powerful diuretic which is used in oedematous conditions to aid in the removal of excess fluid from local areas or body cavities. It is best known, however, for its use in epistaxis in the racehorse — a purpose for which it is banned in this country.

The purpose of this section is to provide basic information on the type of drug used in clinical equine conditions. The list described is only a specimen of what is available.

Most drugs are restricted to professional use for very good reason. However, the horse-owner of today wants information about what is being done and why.

Do not be afraid to ask your veterinary surgeon to enlighten you. He will be only too glad to oblige.

Index

Page numbers *in italics* refer to illustrations

201